Milk & Meditation: Loving Self through Cancer and Chemo

Reverend Suzanne Winterton, D.Div. B.Ed.

ISBN 978-0-244-20522-5

Milk & Meditation:
Loving Self through Cancer and Chemo

For our ever supportive friends:

'Your love has kept (us) going...' [Diana Ross]

Also by Suzanne Winterton:

Life's Veiled Mystery, lulu.com. 2012

Living Spirituality, lulu.com. 2012

Lifting Life's Veil, lulu.com. 2012

Chakras with Love, lulu.com. 2015

Sputnik's Lore: Accepting Ourselves, lulu.com. 2015

The Arrow and the Song:

'I shot an arrow into the air,
It fell to earth, I knew not where;
For, so swiftly it flew, the sight
Could not follow it in its flight.

I breathed a song into the air,
It fell to earth, I knew not where;
For who has sight so keen and strong,
That it can follow the flight of song?

Long, long afterward, in an oak
I found the arrow, still unbroke;
And the song, from beginning to end,
I found again in the heart of a friend.'

Henry Wadsworth Longfellow

Introduction – Holding The Mirror

Suzanne had just enjoyed her 61st birthday. Although an enjoyable day, it had not been quite the celebration that her husband, Garry, had arranged for her 60th. Then, he'd booked Lincoln Guildhall for a formal 'black tie' dinner to which they'd invited friends who'd played a significant role in her life to date; the personal meal - enjoyed at the historic table, decorated with City of Lincoln silverware and adorned with freesias - was memorably concluded with a speech where she gave each guest meaningful acknowledgment, and ended with a quotation attributed to Bletchley code breaker Alan Turing: *'Sometimes it is the people no one can imagine anything of who do the things no one can imagine.'*

An ordinary English woman, Suzanne had already accomplished unimaginable things: she'd left a promising teaching career to follow an inner imperative to be a healer, to guide others in meditation, and to write books about metaphysics.

In her late thirties she'd successfully come through severe clinical depression, for which she'd been hospitalised and given a series of electro shock treatments. She and Garry had been told that she would spend the rest of her life needing to be treated for the illness, and that she must always take anti-depressants, but she'd dismissed the advice, and by using meditation, had become free from all medication.

She'd thought that mental illness was her 'thing' to conquer through life, and was proud of her success. So it was with utter disbelief that she discovered a large lump in her left breast...

Two weeks later, upon receiving the shocking diagnosis of breast cancer, her everyday life – and Garry's – was turned upside down; their days became dominated by hospital appointments, treatments, side-effects, surgery...all happening under the emotional cloud of cancer.

During the early weeks of treatment Suzanne lost a few friendships – presumably those who were unable to deal with the challenge that cancer presents – but gained a closeness with others who found individual ways of supporting her and Garry.

This nucleus of friends became recipients of emails that Suzanne wrote almost daily; for her, writing was cathartic; often she awoke with a song playing through her mind, and realised the lyrics were a particular support through the dark days of experiencing the effects of chemo treatment.

Sharing these lyrics, and receiving loving responses from friends, 'kept her going', and some suggested that she ought to spread her thoughts more widely by making her collection of emails into a book...

'Milk & Meditation: Loving Self through Cancer and Chemo' takes its title from two modes of 'healing' during chemo treatment: **meditation** enabled Suzanne to maintain a sense of peace throughout the ordeal; **milk** became an effective remedy for 'chemo nausea' – it was discovered in the early hours of a morning while a patient in Fraser ward,

Nottingham City hospital: in the darkness, nurse Kim, having listened to Suzanne's distressed misery, gently suggested, "Why not try milk?" Thereafter, every early hours 'side-effects waking' was immediately assuaged by a bowl of Rice Krispies soaked in cold milk.

Suzanne - and Garry – will be forever in Kim's debt for giving them an effective tool to deal with months of night-time distress.

And they both appreciate the loving compassion of oncology nurses, specialists, and technicians whose combined expertise was ready for their need.

This book celebrates their work, and hopefully will be inspirational for all who read it.

Suzanne Winterton. April 2019.

Holding the mirror:

The role of the wounded healer: to deeply know what it's like - not only to have sensitive compassion, but true empathy.

'Oh she takes care of herself, she can wait if she wants

She's ahead of her time

Oh, she never gives out and she never gives in

She just changes her mind…

But, she's always a woman to me.' [Joel]

'Free to decide what matters to you and what never will; whose opinion you value and whose you can disregard, and what exactly is worth your precious hours on this earth and what is a waste of damn time. And really, what could be more beautiful than that.' **[Benedetta Barzini in** *Vogue* **July 2018]**

1 Discovery

March 18th 2018. My birthday. 61 today! A wonderful day: movie theatre at *Kinema In the Woods*, Woodhall Spa, to see, *Peter Rabbit*. Gifts: flowers, an *Alexa show*, and a fun toy remote-controlled Mini to wizz around our living room! Evening meal of pizza with the children we care for, who live across the road.

Monday, March 19th. A creative day; after writing intensely on the manuscript of my sixth book, I leaned back with satisfaction and rested my hand against my breast. I felt a lump. **'What is this?'** - about 3 cm, feeling soft, hadn't noticed it before. It must be a cyst.

I went to Garry in the TV room: "Don't want to worry you, but I can feel a lump, here in my left breast…"

He shrugged his shoulders as I apologised for my usual psychosomatic imaginings.

Wednesday, March 20th. Sitting in Lincoln Cathedral, waiting for the weekly intercessor prayer group meeting that I'd joined two years previously, I gazed up at the stained glass image of Jesus, his arm outstretched in healing, and murmured, 'healing for me, please; healing for me, healing for me, please'.

At the prayer meeting I hinted of a potential problem to Canon Michael, and later that afternoon told my hairdresser, Rosa. She compassionately wagged her finger at me, "You go and see a doctor…it can be just a tiny place in the breast…they give a little tablet to take each day…it'll be fine!"

Late that evening, just before bed, panic set in when Garry felt the lump; we spoke to our closest neighbour by 'phone, and her husband - a doctor - murmured across our conversation: if it's cancer, age is on my side…

An inner scream erupted somewhere inside my head: **'You can't talk about cancer. Not with me. It's not possible.'**

Thursday, March 21st. An 8am call to the medical practice…no doctors available, so we accepted an appointment with a nurse; she examined my breast and hinted that a cyst would be drained; she left us waiting in her office while she went to consult a doctor! He made a routine referral to Nottingham Breast Institute…

During the two-week wait for a breast care appointment, each day is surreal: disbelief; body trembles; tired and thirsty; push food around my plate… I ruminate: it must be a cyst – no cancer has ever manifest in the females of my family; it will be a cyst, but if it's cancer I'll happily accept surgery and radiotherapy, but *not* chemo.

I'm not afraid of dying, but want to live – so much enjoyment, what a waste of this life if I'm to leave now; surely there's greater opportunity of fulfilment for me? I've always loved owning nice things. What's the point in shopping now?

I clear out stuff from my wardrobe…won't need long dresses…ever again.

While Garry is at work I scream at the ceiling, 'Don't want Garry to be in grief, don't want Garry to be in grief, don't want Garry to be in grief… Please help him.'

Each night, I sleep really well, but upon waking have to start the mind calming again…

For years I've lived with the same depressive first thought of the day – it's my dark companion: 'Oh God, another morning, I don't want it'... But now its morbid presence is doubly unwelcome; my mind's unruly habit has to *stop*, because *I do want the day, I do, I do.*

My daily meditative work is maintained: letting go of negative thoughts and emotions, breath-work and mantras, as well as beautiful images; I'm thankful that I learned the practice years ago – meditation has been the 'staple diet' for my mind for so long, and now comes naturally, especially upon waking and before sleep.

I contemplate unusual thoughts that have been on my mind over recent months:

If the next 20 years are like this - days out, shopping, money, eating out, being in the lovely home - *it's not enough.*

If I died after just this loveliness, my life would be unfulfilled.

Is my meditative work truly important for the world?

Is there really purpose in what I do?

Is creative writing all that's in store for me?

Then I wonder: Why, in the writing of my second psychological/spiritual novel, did I decide that one of the characters should develop breast cancer?! I'd resisted the nagging idea because I love the character and didn't want her to suffer! And I was also aware that I couldn't write about breast cancer with realism...

Be careful what you wish for.

I recall inexplicable decisions made over the last few weeks: to withdraw from voluntary work, to cancel the meditation group, to make a new website video, to stop accompanying the children to swimming, to end work at the Cathedral. Why?

What am I to do now?

Wisdom tells me: *How we think and feel is up to us.*

I decide that *it's up to me* to change the way I think and feel... I'm sure that readjusting thought and emotion is part of my healing...

I must undo feelings of **resentment**, as well as **anger** and **disappointment**; these unpleasant judgmental emotions actually accompany profound *love* – the loving hope that friends and clients will use wisdom to make the best decisions for themselves; and whatever I perceive as a disconnection between me and others needs to be corrected, so that I may calm the frustration of being misunderstood.

I must let go of grief, anxiety and fear, as well as regret.

I need to fully accept my self-giving spiritual nurturance.

I have thoughts that the diagnosis is worse than I imagine.

I am not my thought...

Fill each thought with *light*.

Fill the day with *light*.

Inspire it...

Improved thoughts ought to mean that cancer is moved out and away, and so I hold an assertive conversation with the diseases that haunt me: 'Cancer and depression – neither of you are helpful to my body, but I am inspired by your presence. Inspiration continues, and will continue forever. Therefore, it's time for both of you to leave, be out of me, out of my consciousness.'

Healing thoughts influence my body:

I imagine there's a block at second chakra – like a cholesterol obstruction; thought targets my spine: I think about red rising more easily, flowing up through my body; this is a gradual clearing and cleansing, and I thank my body for its helpful activity.

Since there's a lump in my breast, there must be a blockage here too; it's likely to be emotional resistance – that I've wanted to love, to gift to others who are not able to receive healing love. As the block is released there is free flow of wisdom, allowing me to love, and give, without concern of where goodness flows...

Love flows from me, from every part of me, like a mountain stream; where others cannot receive, the love continues unrestricted, flowing wherever it wills...

5

Garry and I spend the Easter weekend in Cambridge; as we walk the beautiful streets sometimes I feel uplifted and positive, then I find myself watching people, scanning their faces…as I did when I was deeply depressed.

I feel waves of sadness, grief, disbelief, and pain that I'm leaving all this, and leaving Garry. What will he do, on his own? I don't want him to be in pain, in grief; I can't bear for him to suffer.

Eventually I steel myself to read the information from Nottingham City hospital regarding clinic procedures. I feel terror: I cannot go there for the examination, then wait for a week, in mental torture, to return for the 'results clinic' – I just can't…

April 5th 2018. We drive to Nottingham Breast Cancer Institute, and find the staff welcoming, sensitive and kind.

Sitting in the waiting room I imagine sending healing energy to other women, clearing the rooms of negativity, and sending good energy into the examination rooms and to the people who work there.

I cry before the mammogram; but as I lay on my side for the ultrasound my tears are under control…

Then the doctor announced she was about to do a biopsy.

"But this is a cyst, right?"

"No, this is a lump."

Her words ought to have brought renewed panic, but instead an overwhelming wave of relaxed calm ripples through my body.

With eyes closed I murmur to Garry seated in the corner of the room, "Are you alright?"

He had sight of the screen - of cancerous lumps in breast and lymph nodes, "I'm here."

We're immediately assigned a breast cancer nurse; she knew exactly how to manage our reactions; she affirmed that there was cancer, and spoke gently and firmly, "This does not necessarily mean you will die sooner."

Her words don't immediately sink in, although I felt relief that I'd been spared the week's wait for diagnosis.

For days I think about dying soon.

There is pain, yet joy, being around the neighbour's children, and I'm able to calmly report the news to their mother.

"I thought you'd come to tell me it's a cyst."

I shake my head, wanting to curl up like a baby, and struggle to eat the food she offered.

I don't want our lives, our conversations, to be overwhelmed by a diary of cancer!

April 11th 2018. Our 37th wedding anniversary. We're in London, a two night stay at Claridge's! Room 127 is exquisite – the room number feels just right, but a 7am wakeup from extremely loud external construction work is beyond annoying! Having reported the ongoing noisy interference, we walk Mayfair, hoping that upon our return the hotel management will have resolved the problem.

Inspire… As we stroll the streets I think about inspiring every building, every place, every person…

It's so ironic giving a normal response to each casual greeting:

"How are you?"

"Good, thank you!"

What am I supposed to say?

We are moved to *The Royal Suite - Room 111!*

In the privacy of our own Claridge's sitting room I play the piano, and then, when our guest, Alan, arrives, Garry requests that our butler serves afternoon tea for three; we're strangely at home in the hotel's grandest rooms!

April 12th 2018. Awake at 4am, amazed to be spending the night in The Royal Suite, in a bed where Royals and Heads of State have slept.

There's a pulsating pain through my breast – a psychosomatic reaction to my anxiety, my quashed terror.

Light shines through my crown; it greets the light of my heart, becoming a combination of Light of me and Light of God.

'Breathe on me breath of God…'

I *inspire* my body.

I welcome *Love,* as Light, to enter through my crown and fill my whole being.

My body is a lighted beacon, shining out love; love for myself, and love for others to be attracted to, and to feel.

As the day unfolds I behave in a surprisingly normal way – as a healthy person, a private guest in Claridge's Royal Suite! I ask the butler to pack all our complementary goodies so that we can enjoy them later in Nottingham – at the Breast Clinic where we are to meet the consultant for confirmation of cancer. I tell myself I will return here, to Claridge's, cured and healed.

Claridge's staff wish us a wonderful day, and apologise again for our initial disturbance; they tell us our day can only get better...

Well...not the kind of day that we face...

There's a sensitive response from Tim, duty manager, and Glenn, manager in the restaurant, who rushes to shake my hand as we leave, "Good Luck."

Their 'thinking of you' card arrived a day later. Thank you.

'From the sublime to ridiculous' is how I describe our drive from Claridge's Hotel, London, to Nottingham, to attend the results clinic.

My initial calm turns to a despairing impatient desire

to walk out after 1 ½ hour wait. Garry sensed my panic and, surprisingly for him, instructed me to meditate – to find my inner garden…

I close my eyes and visualized myself in a beautiful garden where I 'see' myself being greeted by *applauding Angels!*

Thinking I need to follow a path from the garden to a beach, I'm surprised to find myself seemingly *at the summit of a high mountain, and soon feel calmly exhilarated with each meditative breath.*

Ego assured, I face the surgeon and calmly and assertively tell him I want to work with him, but will not accept chemo. He glanced nervously at the attending nurse and made it clear that my *only option for treatment was chemo first, followed by surgery and radiation, and then, maybe Herceptin.*

My strong centre collapsed, and I felt faint. As the consultant left to allow us to process the news and make our decision, I curled up on the couch like a wounded foetus.

Garry had done his research; he spoke with honesty, clarity and wisdom: for me to be with him, to stay with him, it was essential to accept chemo, "You don't start a job with only a few tools to hand."

Immediately, I agreed.

Comment:

'Cancer of the breast must have a special significance for one who has been nurturing so many. You are surely right in feeling that you have much to do. Many people need you and your inspiration, and your determination will bring you through to a greater future for them, and for you and Garry. Congratulations for achievements past and future. Please give my love and thanks to Garry.

I greatly admire the way in which you healed your life by healing others. There is no doubt that you have given much. I pray that you will receive the healing which you so deserve and that you will grow as a result. You gave me so much during the period of our therapeutic connection. You still do.' Alan

2 Support Established

Friday, April 13th 2018

A good day.

Garry and I had discussed whether we tell friends and neighbours: an interesting conundrum – if, for example, I'd suddenly manifested something like a 'personal itch' we would not let it be known, wouldn't dream of talking about it, so why think that breast cancer should be announced? To some, and not to others?

We make the decision to tell a few in the spirit of authenticity, and because we value their love.

So, we invite close neighbours to separate coffee dates…

Their response was the same: shock; overwhelming love expressed with tight, warm hugs; affirmation of support; loving care for Garry; positive thoughts.

So, having done all disclosures considered necessary, we have *our local support...*

Garry chooses to tell just a few at work.

Each day now must unfold as it wills...

An early morning walk with J, children and dogs: slipping into clothes, and out quickly into the day, is helpful.

A drive to Lincoln to get Juanita, my VW Beetle, 'MOT' passed: I'd always believed myself to be mindful, but today I appreciate the joy of driving, with patient detachment of others' ill-mannered behaviour, knowing I'd get to my destination on time.

A phone call from *oncology* department: taken with amazing calmness as I peruse the diary - for Tuesday April 17th at 11.30.

A meet-up with Garry for coffee: seated in the coffee shop our conversation is like friends getting together for a catch-up; his words, still with the same wise focus he'd shown at hospital, now with a willingness to talk about thoughts and emotions – a different Garry from former years!

We discuss the reaction of others: his boss is knowledgeable having a sister-in-law who has just been successfully treated for similar cancer; Dad's main concern is that he'll lose our attention as his carers; Garry's Mother copes with the shock by offering substantial monies if private healthcare is needed.

A shopping spree in TK Maxx for spunky hats is fun! I buy them to affirm that *I* decide upon my future appearance...

A spritely walk to hairdresser, Rosa, to tell her of the confirmation of cancer, and to ask her to do my hair – "Number 2 all over, please!" With classic Italian verve, she shrugs her shoulders, "Yes! We'll shave your hair... Other clients have done the same. You, Suzanne, are so strong and positive."

How do people perceive strength in me, when I've always felt afraid?

A march up Steep Hill to the Cathedral. I wonder whether to leave a prayer request card at the altar – prayers of thanks for Garry, and for healing... As I consider what to write, I think about how my card will be read by the group that I've come to know; they'll learn about cancer from my prayer, and realise I'll be absent from the weekly meetings...

I pause, unable to construct a written prayer. Suddenly, the Cathedral environment feels...barren. I gaze at my favourite stained glass image of Jesus reaching his hand to the lame man; then I light a candle – with my usual whispered prayer: 'for my family, the whole world' - and happily leave... Little knowing a year will pass before I return.

At home, I wonder why I've been searching supermarkets for good quality *mango juice*. After 'Googling' the query, I'm thrilled at the first note: mango juice benefits those with breast cancer! There's a childish delight in my smile: *me and my body are in touch!*

I choose the menu, cook our dinner, and *eat!*

During an evening coffee discussion, our neighbour recalls how our arrival in the village had brought people together; her husband said the cancer was a way for me to show something special; I agreed, but spoke of feeling abandoned - that I'd not seen the usual images of Angels and Jesus; he scratched his chin, thoughtfully, "That reminds me of the verse called, 'Footprints': when you see only one set of footprints, that's the time when *you are being carried."*

Oh, God. I love.

I have my first Reiki treatment:

When the session began I could smell frankincense, even though there was none in the oil diffuser.

During the treatment my right index finger kept spontaneously moving – as it did during hypnotherapy; I think of it as communication of my subconscious mind being part of the process and affirming each part of the therapy; I was glad to feel it.

I felt a sudden sharp pain through my left breast; it felt 'good'. Then, as the work continued over my heart chakra, I imaged a pyramid hovering over my chest.

I felt tingling across my arms and breast.

About half way through the session I imaged a separation of parts of myself – as if my 'etheric' body had lifted itself away from my 'physical' body, so that work could be done, just on the physical.

There was a tingling sensation through base chakra.

At the end of the work, as her hands pressed against the soles of my feet, I felt that the etheric had descended back into place; I moved my arms above my head, appreciating the energy movement through my body.

At some point I remember using the mantra, 'Let go, let God...' and I recall thanking the consciousness of cancer for its presence – teaching me wisdom.

I affirmed that I would continue to pursue this wisdom, and confirmed that cancer should now depart from me, my body, my consciousness.

'And so it is.'

Afterwards, I felt calm, peaceful and refreshed.

My therapist said she perceived a mass at my throat, 'like frog spawn', and thought that it meant I had 'a lot to say'. She perceived a large, red English rose at my heart, and saw an image of a ring, having a deep red stone within. She felt energy travelling up and down the core of my body.

I'm grateful for all the healing I am receiving. Thank you.

I remember friendships that, over the years, have broken down; and, being aware of the mind/body connection, think about how this fragmentation will have contributed to my dis-ease; I decide to create an 'Outspoken Thought' of what I ought to say to people I've not spoken with for some time, yet have not forgotten; even though my words will not be consciously read, the sentiment is communicated in thought, and writing is healing:

I write about how resentment and judgment have been unpleasant personality traits for me to wrestle with; how I give, and love, deeply but conditionally, which means that when I feel and see things that I judge to be 'not right', I'm profoundly disappointed; I know that this mistaken behaviour is harmful to me and everyone else.

In my mind, I invite former friends to come close to me...as close as they can:

'**Come into my heart** - *the place that does not harbour thought and emotion, the place that is the real me. As you enter, please join with me to send away every thought, every emotion, everything that has stood between us...*

RESENTMENT

RESENT

RE-SENT

Everything that is not good for us, is re-sent back to 'God'.

'God' – Pure Consciousness - is, by its nature, receiving of everything; changing wounds into unwounded. Where I fail, It draws through me with unconditional love.

It sets us free from unpleasantness.

As our hearts nestle, we are whole. Love, Suzanne'

I think about friends and clients who've had breast cancer, and search documents to find commentaries of their healing sessions. I'm glad to read and recall how we worked, how images and songs came together for their healing, how we hoped that invasive treatment would not be necessary, but in the event of chemo and radiation being needed, affirmed that healing complements the skills of medics.

I send love to them – those now in spirit and those embodied.

Comment:

'Dear Suzanne,

I can understand you must feel devastated. I HOPE YOU WILL ALSO FEEL VALUED AND ENHANCED. I was asking the I Ching yesterday what will be best for you. It gave hexogram 8, Holding Together: *'Holding together brings good fortune. What is required is that we unite with others, in order that all may complement and aid one another through holding together. But such holding together calls for a central figure around which other people may unite. To become a centre of influence, holding people together, is a grave matter and fraught with great responsibility. It requires greatness of spirit, consistency and strength. Therefore let him who wishes to gather others about him ask himself whether he is equal to the undertaking,'* YES, SUZANNE, YOU ARE EQUAL TO THE CHALLENGE *'for anyone attempting the task without a real calling for it only makes confusion worse than if no union at all had taken place. But when there is a real rallying point, those who at first are hesitant or uncertain gradually come in of their own accord.'*

When I asked again just now, what you should do, I was given hexogram 45, Gathering Together: *'Gathering together. Success. The king approaches his temple. It furthers one to see the great man. This brings success. Perseverance furthers. To bring great offerings creates good fortune. It furthers one to undertake something. This describes a man who gathers people around him in the name of the ruler (GOD). Since he is not striving for any special advantages for himself, but is working unselfishly to bring about general unity, his work is crowned with success, and everything becomes as it should be.'*

These answers make it clear that you need to be the central figure in your healing, Suzanne.

You and I, Suzanne, know that you are well equipped to take on this role. In fact it is a role which has come naturally to you in your healing work. In doing so you will be healing not only others, but also yourself. It is a heroic task. You will know how best to do this. I believe you will succeed. More than ever you will be assuming the task of the wounded healer. I wrote already that I find the symbolism of the breast very powerful. WITH GARRY'S HELP, YOU CAN DO IT. MAKE THE DECISION, PRAY FOR THE STRENGTH AND COMMIT YOURSELF ABSOLUTELY TO THE HEALING OF OTHERS. YOUR OWN HEALING WILL COME AS A BY-PRODUCT. I HOPE YOU WILL ALSO WRITE A BOOK, STARTING TODAY. MY THOUGHTS ARE WITH YOU, SUZANNE. THIS IS A GREAT CHALLENGE. I BELIEVE YOU WILL TRIUMPH. PLEASE FEEL FREE TO CALL ME AT ANY TIME. WITH LOVE AND BLESSINGS,' Alan

'He believes in you like we all do. Strong and meaningful words. I agree, write a book starting today.... xxx'

18

April 14th 2018

My Dad's 93rd birthday. As normal, slept well. Waking is a problem, where disbelief – 'Oh God, the challenge' - is followed by letting go of anxiety and fear using the meditative mantra: *Who Am I, Who Am I, Who Am I'.*

Today, for some reason, I needed to write a piece entitled, *Time for Glands.*

I've little idea about physiology, but the names that come to mind: gonads, adrenal, thymus, thyroid, pituitary, pineal... Each receive instruction, **to be balanced**: balance through receiving red and integrating blue so that my body is swirled with purple.

It was challenging sitting with Dad, listening to him ramble, "Well, you look alright, so you must be... you'll get through this, I'm sure you will... Wear a hat to keep your hair on..."

I feel inexplicably thirsty and hugely tired – how so, since there's no physiological reason?

How do I get through these days so smoothly? Is it that something within takes over? Or that what's happening just doesn't seem real?

Writing becomes very self-motivating; I start sending out thoughts via email – without any creative plan; in fact, songs sound in my head, playing over and over until I acknowledged their presence by writing of them.

3 Curtains Wide

April 15th 2018

'Drinking in the morning sun
Blinking in the morning sun
Shaking off the heavy one
Heavy like a loaded gun...
Throw those curtains wide
One day like this a year'd see me right.' [Elbow]

Dear All,

My healing regime is not 'goal directed' in terms of getting from today, towards a day when someone says, 'clear of cancer';

Rather, this is another day in the life of us, with each day a step forward in learning, growing, loving, being...

There is no 'affirming hoop' to jump through.

This is a smooth journey of mindful steps.

So, when people use the traditional greeting, 'How are you?'

I can truthfully respond, 'I'm good, thank you!'

Love, Suzanne

Dear All,

Cancer is part of the universe.

It has its place: helping many to make their transition; bringing people together; making us see the preciousness of each day.

Cancer, you may feel warm and snug in me; but my breast, my body, is not the rightful place for you. It is no longer necessary for you to remain.

Your purpose here is complete:

It is not time for me to make my transition; people have come together around me; I know the preciousness of each moment of every day.

I, and those around me, speak openly of love, life, dying, living.

I have stepped onto a renewed higher path of healing and spirituality.

All this will continue, forever, without your presence in my being.

Now, you must leave. Leave my body. Be away from my consciousness.

You are commanded to return, completely, to your own place in the universe.

And so it is.

Suzanne

Dear All,

It's time to change language expressions:

What was, 'I have breast cancer', has become, 'My body received a diagnosis of breast cancer; and now, me and my body are healing, returning to perfect balance'.

We learn from news reports how, 'beating this, overcoming that' becomes an escalation of potential war, with each side becoming more obdurate. So, we are not 'beating cancer'; rather, 'we are encouraging, and commanding, cancer to leave, to move on, to return to its own place in the universe'.

This evening it's difficult to understand why my body feels ill: so tired, thirsty, shooting pain through my breast; I feel 'hollow' behind my eyes, and wonder about a comment I'd once heard – that those with cancer have a dark shadow below their eyes... Isn't that just tiredness, or understandable stress?

Don't lose focus, Suzanne; remember your decision: cancer is not the central topic of the day; return to your usual meditative mantra:

'I have a body; a beautiful, amazing body, but I am not my body. Who Am I

I have emotions; a wonderful array of emotions, but I am not my emotions. Who Am I

I have thoughts; billions of thoughts, but I am not my thoughts. Who Am I

I am my Spirit Self. I AM, I AM, I AM.'

Keeping up the fun! Still reeling from the incredulity of being upgraded to the *Royal Suite* at Claridge's, Garry and I decide to watch the DVD documentary about our Mayfair home. There! Nearly the whole programme is devoted to *our* sitting room, *our* entrance, *our* conference room, *our* piano, *our* bed, *our* bathroom, *our* sunken bath! How amazing to have been relocated to Claridge's best!

Suite 111

One. One. One. I am One. Whole. Complete. Loved, and in love with the UNIverse.

Garry and I own the miracle of good sleep, and having worked through shock and horror, we hold on to the miracle of eating.

This morning's miracle: *no wakeup anxiety.* What is this strange normalcy? What do I do now?

Now, you carry on, doing what you do:

Meditate; meditate with breath; meditate noticing each part of your body; smile:

'Throw those curtains wide, one day like this a year'd see me right...'

I asked Garry how I should respond to a neighbour's text: 'How are you both?'

"How are you, Garry?"

"Ok, apart from the elephant in the room."

"There is no elephant."

He raised his eyebrows at George, my teddy bear, "There's a lump in his kapok; but, never mind, he said he'll take chemo!"

What great love is this: that my teddy bear is willing to take on my burden!

Love, Suzanne

Comment:

'Suzanne, your emails are becoming a feature of my day. They're an amazing flow of strength such as I've not experienced before. Really tremendous! Truly wonderful! Thank you, thank you, thank you. Love and gratitude,' Alan

4 Mind & Matter

April 19th 2018

It's a month since I felt the lump in my breast, and a week since the consultant's further news sent me reeling, feeling faint, with the desire to curl up like a foetal baby, in disbelief and additional shock.

So, here we are. We've come through shock, panic, incredulity, grief and despair, to find calm, 'normal' days, facing reality with a focussed plan, determined and strong, with peace-filled purpose.

It's a journey of the process of the mind.

The importance of the *mind* is affirmed by nurses, doctors and almost everyone else, who talk of *the value of thinking positively* after a diagnosis of cancer.

However, when I speak to doctors about healing, and about the *mind/body* connection, their response is usually a wry smile and a shake of the head, which I think means, 'She's slightly crazy, but best not argue.'

I find it disappointing that medical doctors and quantum physicists - both scientists, after all – do not usually agree about the effect of the mind upon the body...with the exception that stress can be seen through physical symptoms.

My oncologist, Dr Chan - being vaguely aware of my metaphysical views - commented that his department could only work with what they understood, but respected the beliefs of others.

Beliefs?

It's not *belief* to know that the Earth is a sphere, nor that we live in one of billions of galaxies.

It's not *belief* that the rise in heart rate, sweating etc. is a physical response to fearful *thoughts and feelings.*

Why is it that, generally, the medical profession is unwilling to consider the *mind and body* connection beyond a physical manifestation of stress?

Where is the boundary between what is *mind influenced* and what is not?

As mankind has made significant and amazing medical progress, the wisdom of centuries old medicine – from the era of Hippocrates - has been dismissed, and laws of physics – realised through Einstein - have not been embraced. And yet, seen together, the work of these two pioneers, confirm psychoneuroimmunology – the mind/body connection.

I learned about Hippocrates – who practiced medicine around 400 BC, and Asclepiades – working around 120 BC, when we spent a Christmas Eve on the island of Kos; there, at the invitation of one of our American friends, we roamed the ancient site of a healing centre where 'modern' medicine began: where massage, spa water, psychological support of patients, analysis of thoughts and dreams, complemented 'revolutionary' ideas of surgery and knowledge of disease. Scientists then knew that *a state of mind changed the state of the body.*

Einstein's Theory of Special Relativity – which includes the famous equation, $E = mc^2$ – tells us that it's mistaken to think of mass as solid when, in fact, matter is made up of vibrating particles and empty space – all of which is energy. Einstein explained that matter – that which we perceive as solid – is energy in a more dense form or slower vibration, making it perceptible to the senses; energy and mass are two facets of the same field, one may be transformed into the other; matter is another form of the same fundamental nature of all life – energy.

Quantum physics shows that ultimately everything in the universe is connected; everything that happens does so because there is an energy making it happen.

Matter is energy…as are thoughts and emotions.

All this knowledge helps us understand the significance of how we feel - that feelings, thoughts and emotions, with differing electromagnetic frequencies, play a vital role in our wellbeing, and the interaction between mind and body determines our state of health.

Hence, the healing of my body (to 'heal' means to make 'whole') is the process of returning to a state of perfect health, by working with energy: changing the energy of thought and emotion, and moving the energy of matter; this, together with surgery and medicine.

During this month, my *physical* symptoms of fear and shock have gone away, and there's been an increased sense of calm. This change happened because of my changed *state of mind*, and because my mind and emotions have found a place of safety. It's true to say that 'time heals' and brings about 'acceptance'; and I think that occasional fearful thoughts that creep into an otherwise peaceful day arise because there is a part of my mind, hiding within, that, despite time's healing, continues to feel terror.

Meditating with the mantra, *'Who Am I'*, is an amazing help. (More about this in a future chapter).

For now, I'd like to end with an image that I think is important for everyone; its aim is to speak to mind, emotion, body and spirit with an encouraging command that each part of ourself is an *equal* aspect of the whole, working together, in shared love and safety; there is no need for any part to feel afraid or abandoned:

Breathing gently, with eyes closed, I find myself in my 'inner garden'; my bare feet luxuriate on the soft grass; I feel warmth from a gentle breeze; my face turns up to the clear blue sky. I know that 'all' of me is here: my physical body, its etheric perfection, emotional self, conscious mind, sub-conscious mind, ego, and spiritual self. All perfect aspects of me. And, as I affirm the presence of all parts of myself, I imagine that we stand in a circle, our arms overlap on each other's shoulders; we're all equal; each part engenders equal respect.

'We' stand, and breathe together. Then, with feet firmly planted on the grass, we lean back from the hips, perfectly balanced and without falling, depending on each other. After a while, we slowly become upright. And then we bend forward from the hips, so that our heads meet in the centre. Eventually, we return to standing upright.

Gradually, 'we' begin to edge forward, closing the circle; each aspect moves at the same pace as all others...slowly closing in...until 'all of me' merges completely. 'We' are one. I am complete with body, mind(s), emotion, spirit.

As 'our' unity becomes total, a bright light descends from above, and shines through so that I am a pillar of light. I'm a beacon in my inner garden: my mind, body, spirit are united. Every part of me feels valued and safe. No part need ever feel alone or afraid. We are together; One.

And so it is.

Love, Suzanne

Comment:

'Dear Suzanne, My! You have been busy, and to such good effect! Every word shows your focus and effectiveness. I'm impressed, Suzanne, deeply impressed. Knowing your thoughts and activities brings me a beautiful, much valued connection. I feel part of your sustaining group, part of your greatness. With love and great respect,' Alan

5 Nature's Way

It's strange to be having a 'normal' day without the busyness of hospitals, or the excitement of birthday, wedding anniversary, and Claridge's! Today's sunshine gives me the first day of the year sitting on the patio; household jobs accomplished, meditation done, I enjoy the twitter of birds, bleating lambs and sheep, garden chimes, and flowing water feature...

My 3-year-old neighbour has been missing his visits to 'Suzanne's house'; his mother had explained to him that I needed to see a doctor for an injection - toddlers are used to injection dramas! He asked me, in quite a serious tone, whether I was feeling better; I assured him I was. He went on to explain how injections have to be given in your leg, they hurt, and make you bleed, but...they make you better.

They do! And, for me, they will do.

However, as I wait for three weeks before chemo begins, I realise that I must 'up the intensity' of meditation. This does not mean trying harder, or thinking more deeply; quite the opposite...

It's about finding *nature's way.*

I've had thoughts about Chernobyl. Some time after the disaster, a news documentary showed how tiny weeds had begun to grow amongst the abandoned concrete; and here, in our country, daisies manage to push up healthy leaves and bright, strong flowers between the cracks of our paths; even by the side of London's tube, buddleia have the ability to produce large shrubs perched precariously in small decaying gutters.

It's Nature's Way – being in touch with itself, and growing without trying.

Meditation is a method of finding Nature's Way...

Setting contemplation aside...and taking a late-in-the-day shower, I feel the lump...it seems bigger and harder...

Tears. *It's an uphill task; what if I fail? What if, after sending positive emails, I fall apart? I'll have let God down. I'll have let Garry down.*

Swiftly moving through the anxiety, telling myself that tearful concern is part of the process, I reaffirm my meditative resolve:

For the last 20 years my day has begun, and ended, with meditation; I've used various strategies – noticing each part of my body; watching thoughts drift through the mind; repeating a mantra; noticing each breath; and using my renowned images that readily spring to mind.

Now, my mind must step aside, completely, so that Nature's Way will flow more easily through me.

So, from today, more frequent times of meditation is the plan – a few minutes set aside to close my eyes, notice each breath, and watch the rise and fall of my abdomen. That's All. It's not easy! Thoughts immediately interrupt, and I find myself off on a thought track without even realising... Then, patiently bring myself back to watching, noticing each breath. When my few minutes is done, I must move on without questioning, or wondering, what I may – or may not – have accomplished. Other forms of meditation will continue, but from now on, strict breath-work is my Nature's Way.

Love, Suzanne

6 I Love You Because

Awake with the voice of Jim Reeves in my head:

'I love you because you understand, dear

Every single thing I try to do

You're always there to lend a helping hand, dear

I love you most of all because you're you

No matter what the world may say about me

I know your love will always see me through

I love you for the way you never doubt me

But most of all I love you 'cause you're you

I love you because my heart is lighter

Every time I'm walking by your side

I love you because the future's brighter

The door to happiness you open wide.' [Jim Reeves]

The lyrics express exactly my relationship with Garry. His steadfast love and constancy rise to another level upon diagnosis of cancer. Our love is the same, but now we give more time to sharing how we feel, and he carefully navigates through each day, managing to remain patient when dealing with the roller-coaster of my emotions.

It's a constant challenge, and occasionally he succumbs to pressure and stress with periodic migraines.

While he rests, there are tears: Why did I do this? Why did this have to happen?

Then my anger vents in silent vicious thought: *'Breast cancer nurse, I don't want to know you. Nottingham volunteer patient support group, I don't want you, don't want to know you, don't want to be part of your xxxx regime; you're useful, but NOT FOR ME. I don't want this, I don't want it...it's not fair...*

I must be rid of this anger, of disappointment and resentment... Let go, let God; let go, let God; let go, let God...

I have to heal this; I have to show the experts that the way forward is to integrate mind/body/spirit therapy with surgery and medicine. I have to show them, I have to show them, I have to show them.'

Dealing with our own feelings is one thing, but we also have to be sensitive to the differing reaction of friends: some actively welcome news about the variety of hospital appointments that flood our diary; but we sense that with others we must say nothing; some people make the decision easy – by choosing to stop communicating altogether! To them I feel a mixture of anger, incredulity, indignation...and compassion.

The diversity of *our* conversational need shows itself even within the space of a few hours of one day: during a spontaneous meet-up for coffee on the patio, neighbours express awe at our continued strength and calmness; whereas, in planned afternoon tea with other friends, we keep to our decision not to disclose our misery. However, after they leave, it feels strangely 'empty' not to have spoken the truth of our situation; my inner confusion and long-term depressive uncertainty is expressed again with what had once been a frequent anxious query, "*Is everything alright?*"

That same sense of 'vacant loss' lurches through me when we walk through town and bump into friends we've not seen in a while; the conversation flowed without mention of cancer since it didn't seem necessary or appropriate to tell them; but afterwards, my bewildered self speaks out: "*Is everything alright? Is this happening? Garry, I can't believe this is happening to me, to us.*"

I'd always declared that I was not afraid of death, but as the reality of cancer seeps through my mind I know I'm in terror of the *process* of dying; when someone speaks to me about death I feel a pang of fear in my gut, and manage to silently gulp away my reaction; but when another person glibly declares, "Well, we've all got to die sometime..." my whole being revolts in anguish: "You speak boldly now, but when *your* moment arrives, you'll feel so very different - inexplicably different."

*However close one has been to 'death', in whatever circumstance one has experienced grief and mourning, our thought is never ready for when dying applies to **us**. **But, when we come face to face with our own 'mortality'...and find 'recognition'...it becomes the making of us.***

Indeed, one wise friend affirms my most profound thought: that breast cancer is a journey for me, a learning journey that I will safely come through.

Who better to make this journey, than me?

Days of abnormal calm are interspersed with the return of my life-long habit of waking-up feeling nauseous, and now with various psychosomatic pains; it's good that I've not yet started chemo as I would have blamed my symptoms on the treatment. I have a sneaking fear that the cancer may be worse than first thought.

The surprise and shock of 'me with cancer' keeps returning, making me feel disconnected: Is this really the body I've always known? What did I miss? How did I not know? Having cancer present in my body does not seem 'real'.

We talk about it, but it can't be *true*...

...Then there's good sleep and calm waking, even a Saturday morning sleep-in followed by a leisurely breakfast; things that are simple and normal for others, bring me much appreciation and joy.

The emotional roller-coaster continues amidst frequent appointments at Nottingham City Hospital: MRI, ECG, blood tests, lesson about chemo with questionnaires, a 'marker' inserted in the centre of the lump so that its original size and location is clear for whenever chemo causes it to shrink or disappear...

Tell the car, 'Nottingham' - it'll know where to go!

What was once, 'I don't want chemo', is now an urgent desire to get started, even eager anticipation...

Some phone calls from the hospital are received with mature calmness, others cause me to literally feel weak at the knees - such as the call from a 'trials' nurse' who tells me of 'good news'. (I hadn't been aware that the news was especially 'bad'). In fact, a borderline laboratory test result, that had been re-checked in Edinburgh, confirms that my body will work with Herceptin, so we're invited for yet another hospital visit to affirm that I'll be part of a research trial.

Each trip to Nottingham has to include a shopping expedition with a determination to seek out anything exotic: purple painted toenails, expensive perfume, extreme coloured lipstick, clothes that I don't need, but must have... Garry and I share the desire to complement each hospital escapade with an 'escape treat', and in receiving, I tell my body, *'You did really well today.'*

Then, amidst all the emotional challenges, there's an amazing event: while at the wheel of my lovely cabriolet Beetle, sitting in the sunshine in a queue of traffic, I *have* to say to myself, **'I feel happy'.**

'The tranquilly balanced soul. Rooted in the warmth of affection, elegance flowers in creative expression, like a mountain ascending through brilliance to the heights of heaven.' [I Ching of the Goddess]

Comment:

'Dear Suzanne, It's wonderful how you manage this difficult time and keep going. *An end is always followed by a new beginning.'* Alan

7 Venn Diagram

During the years of working through depression, whenever I was out walking through crowds, I used to scan people's faces...searching... I'd no idea why, or what I was hoping to achieve; it was never a good activity, it always made me feel sad and lonely.

Now, I've returned to the same habit: I find myself watching women, wondering if they have breast cancer, wondering what they, and the man holding their hand, are feeling; I also notice the behaviour of youngsters...and focus my attention on them...wondering what their health future holds...

Perhaps, years ago, I was *soul searching*, looking for some kind of recognition.

Now, with each thought connection, I send each person Love.

As usual, during my morning shower, I think about how much I love my body – and tell it so:

Massaging shower gel over my skin, I murmur, 'You're beautiful...every part of you is beautiful; arms and hands, fingers and scalp...you're wonderful; breasts and tummy, hips and legs...however you're feeling, I know you're amazing; important little places...you're lovely! Face and head...you glow with refreshing water, I love you; back and spine...you're so strong, I appreciate your power; dear skin...all over me, you're incredible.'

Towelling dry, and treating my skin to luxurious body lotion, I murmur similar loving phrases, and then, with my own form of self-reflexology, I sit and massage my feet, repeating a mantra: *'Father God, Earth Mother; Father God, Earth Mother; Father God, Earth Mother.'*

Nevertheless, today there's another emotional 'blip' with the persistent return of resentment, disappointment, frustration and anger; I have to keep on, keeping on, healing the thought patterns and correcting my judgmental personality trait.

After years of researching metaphysical topics, I've come to understand that the energy of emotions naturally resides in the second chakra – in the pit of the stomach. It's obvious! Right there I feel the churn of anxiety and the boil of anger!

The frequent use and abuse of unpleasant emotions – feelings that have become my close companions at the expense of love and patience - means that unhealthy energy cycles through me and sediments into my body; I'm certain that resentment, disappointment, frustration and anger are unhealthy, and where they linger, lodged in and around me, they have the potential of being the 'death' of me.

I'm resolved to turn away from this existence, and instead, firmly choose 'life's wisdom': to live in peace, with patience, understanding, allowing, acceptance – in effect, I choose Healing Love.

An image of a Venn diagram comes to mind: emotions rest in a circle, and Healing Love has its circle too; unhelpful emotions collect in one circle; higher choice emotions in another; Healing Love circle is the third.

The circles gradually merge, closer and closer, until they are one.

Healing Love subsumes all – that is its nature, its purpose, its power. The completed glowing circle becomes a sphere, a cell-like traveller, living in my body, moving through every part of me, subsuming all that is unhealthy with Healing Love.

And so it is. Love, Suzanne

Comment:

'Gentle success through what is small in advancing and in retreating. The will wavers. The perseverance of a warrior furthers.'
Alan

8 The Point

Awake. What day is it? Monday. Today we're to have a meal out, so no need to think about what food to prepare.

Our lunch companions don't need to know about____; that's good.

What clothes do I need? What colour?

Ok, got the plan...

Meditate: notice each part of my body, then watch breath and breathing, and use a mantra, 'Father God, Earth Mother...'

Watch the beautiful sky...

Now it's possible to get out of bed, and be in the day.

This has been my 'getup' strategy for years - sometimes more effective than others:

'Some days are diamonds, some days are stones

Sometimes the hard times won't leave me alone

Sometimes a cold wind blows a chill in my bones

Some days are diamonds, some days are stones.' [Denver]

There's nothing to write today.

Will they be pleased to have no email from me?

What's the point?

If there's not a point, then there is no point.

This is not a depressive wail. It's about finding the *reason for being.*

My mind goes back 15 years...to a morning when my parents joined Garry and me for 'coffee and news'. My Mother sighed with satisfaction as she sat down and removed her scarf, "**We** have a grandson!"

My stomach lurched, and my self-centred ego blurted, "What about me? What have I done that's worthwhile?"

She glanced around our sunroom, and smiled, "Oh, you have a lovely home!"

My heart seemed as if it would explode into a million pieces: Is my home all that I am? Is my life just about the good things around me?

I felt crushed...by jealousy, and by being misunderstood.

It's true: Garry and I have always been project minded; for 38 years there's always been something, 'on the go'; our philosophy wasn't planned; the ideas flow naturally; the point was not to be materially minded, but to create niceness around us as a way of nurturing each other – of expressing love. *That's the point.*

When the diagnosis of cancer gripped my consciousness, I felt crushed again as I looked around our home: 'What's the point? Why do we have this? Why have we created such beauty, to have it dashed in such a short time? Why didn't I see 'the end' coming? Why wasn't I prepared? Where are Angels when I need them most?

My scream erupted out aloud, into the echo of our living room: 'I don't want him to be alone, I don't want him to be alone, I don't want him to suffer, I don't want him to be in grief, please help him, please draw close and be with him.'

What's the point?

The point has been - to share myself, my life; and in that sharing, he and I are happy.

However, there is another point.

When I began these musings, I wrote that our life, as good as it is, did not seem enough.

My words found 'inspiration' – inspire, breathe into everything, filling with love…creating fulfilment.

Finding the point.

What's the source of inspiration and fulfilment?

Where's the point?

I recall a meditative image that appeared a week ago:

As I focussed on breathing, noticing each breath,

I saw a line, a strong beam, across my shoulders;

another line, a strong beam, appeared across my hips;

the two beams were joined by lines down each side of my body;

*I was enclosed in a **square**.*

*Another shape appeared inside the square – a **triangle**;*

its base across my hips,

its apex at my throat;

*within the triangle, there was a **circle**, squashed into an ellipse.*

As I breathed, and watched, the shapes became three dimensional:

a cube, contained a pyramid, with a conical sphere within.

The shapes did not seem to offer meaning;

*but suddenly, with a feeling of euphoria, I perceived **what's inside**…*

A tiny dot, right in the centre,

like a minute blue pearl, deep within, throbbing with beauty.

That's It.

That's the point.

Lunch with friends feels somehow surreal; once again, the usual greeting of, 'How are you?' holds much significance, and it seems odd not to respond with truth, especially when the question is repeated.

At the end of a pleasant meal I excuse myself and, upon my return, it's clear the atmosphere has changed: Garry had taken the opportunity to update our companions... Their seemingly nonchalant response somehow feels encouraging.

As the day draws to a close, it's strange to keep feeling pain through both breasts; I'm thirsty and tired...

Lots of tears: tomorrow we go to meet the oncologist...I'm frightened. *'Take this cup away from me, for I don't want to taste its poison.'* [Jesus Christ Superstar]

Breathe.

This can't be happening to me. I'm revolted and reviled at the thought of allowing poison into me. I'm sorry body; I'm so sorry. You can rise through this – Chernobyl did...

Mindfully I fold my beautiful laundry, and mindfully fold Garry's - caring for both of us.

'I have a body, but I am not my body...'

I've used poison before: tranquilisers, anti-depressants, shock treatment... My body withstood then; my body has worked with me before; my body came through perfectly, beautifully.

It is beautiful now, and will continue to be.

Comment:

'I'm sure that Garry is giving unstinting support and you

know that you have the concern and prayers of your friends. So, however difficult it may be, the watchwords are surely: onward and upward. Very best wishes for successful treatment of those 'pesky cells': they don't know what's about to hit them!!' R

9 Who Am I

I'm preoccupied with sickening thoughts: concern at how my body will react to chemo, and terror of cancer taking over my body if I don't have the treatment.

When the two-sided fear overwhelms me, I find calm by repeating: '*I have a body, but I am not my body; I have a body, but I am not my body*'.

This therapeutic phrase actually evolved from a meditative mantra:

'*Who Am I*'

Who am I

The three words are not meant to be a question, nor a rhetorical expression; they're simply a fundamental method of meditating.

Sri Ramana Maharshi, a well-respected guru, suggested that, '*Who Am I*' is the only mantra necessary for effective meditation.

Years ago I took his teaching seriously, and have greatly benefitted from using, '*Who Am I*' in my meditative practice.

In fact, 'Who Am I' effectively carried me through the initial horror of cancer diagnosis, and using this form of meditation could save many from painful thoughts and emotions that are so destructive in everyday life.

(I've previously written how, *noticing one's breath* is *the* meditative way of stopping the mind's chattering stream of thought; however, dedicated meditators soon discover that thoughts are clever in their persistence, and in order to rein them in it's necessary to use varying methods of meditation - noticing each part of one's body, watching breathing, noticing thoughts, repeating a mantra, creating peaceful images.)

Roberto Assagioli - a psychiatrist with particular interest in transpersonal psychology – effectively expanded, 'Who Am I' into a profound meditational piece:

I have a body, but I am not my body; who am I

I have emotions, but I am not my emotions; who am I

I have thoughts, but I am not my thoughts; who am I

The phrases are therapeutic:

Where my body may be disfigured through surgery; and where my body may suffer during cancer treatment...

Or, where there is dislike of the body's appearance...

I have a body, but I am not my body; who am I

I have a body, but I am not my body; who am I

The repeated phrase adjusts the mistaken belief that our physical body is, 'who we are', and calms our anguish.

Where emotions of fear, anxiety, grief, resentment, overpower the way I feel...

Or, where we mistakenly claim ownership of feelings: '*I* am angry', '*I* am frightened'...

I have emotions, but I am not my emotions; who am I

I have emotions, but I am not my emotions; who am I

The repeated phrase takes away our preoccupation with the way we feel, and releases the mistaken belief that our feelings determine, 'who we are'.

Where thoughts race through my mind, scattering peaceful order...

Or, where thoughts have the power to make us believe we are 'bad'...

I have thoughts, but I am not my thoughts; who am I

I have thoughts, but I am not my thoughts; who am I

The repeated phrase dismisses our concern with whatever we think, and corrects our idea that thoughts make us, 'who we are'.

The meditation is mind-changing!

After I received the cancer diagnosis, whenever I've wanted to cry about what has happened, and what may happen, to my body, 'Who Am I' brings peace.

Whenever I've found myself shaking with fear, 'Who Am I' makes me calm.

Whenever I realise I'm thinking morbid thoughts, 'Who Am I' creates purpose.

My meditation combines Maharshi and Assagioli:

*I have a body; a wonderful, amazing physical body; I have a body that knows exactly how to be its natural self; I have a beautiful body that carries me around throughout this lifetime; I have a body, but I am **not** my body; Who Am I*

*I have emotions; an amazing array of emotions that I use to express myself; I have emotions, but I am **not** my emotions; Who Am I*

*I have thoughts; billions of thoughts through day and night; thoughts that I use to construct my perceptions of life; I have thoughts, but I am **not** my thoughts; Who Am I*

I AM

I AM

I AM

Please use this way of meditating for yourself.

Love, Suzanne

10 Colour Me

Awake, with two verses going round and round in my mind; the words become a desperate repetition, trying to settle the 'butterflies' as we prepare for a day of major appointments at Nottingham City Hospital; this time: for a 'marker' to be placed in the tumour so that its original location can be verified whenever it's time for surgery; an MRI; and...we're to meet the oncologist.

First, my mind replays phrases from, *'A Course in Miracles'...*

'A Course in Miracles [ACIM] is a 1976 manual containing a curriculum which claims to assist its readers in achieving spiritual transformation. The underlying premise of the work is the teaching that the greatest 'miracle' that one may achieve in one's life is the act of simply gaining a full 'awareness of love's presence'. The book was written, or 'scribed', by Helen Schucman, who claimed that it had been dictated to her word for word via 'inner dictation' which came from Jesus.' [Wikipedia]

I studied the 'Course' some years ago, and found its daily phrases transformed my way of thinking from 'needy' to self-empowering.

My waking thought has two statements in mind:

ACIM 67: 'Love created me like itself.'

ACIM 361: *'This Holy Instant would I give to You. Be you in charge. For I would follow You, certain that Your direction gives me peace.'*

Lots of tears: I've lost focus; my thought has been wandering...worrying about chemo, about my body, about side-effects...

Mustn't let myself drift from healing; keep to the *real* strategy:

Let go of negative thoughts;

release unhealthy emotions;

do what comes naturally:

'Let your love flow, like a mountain spring

Let your love grow, with the smallest of dreams

Let your love bind you to all living things

Let your love shine, and you'll know what I mean

It's the reason.' [Bellamy Brothers]

As we drive to Nottingham, I talk about the wonderful circumstance – that for years, unknown to us, an oncology department has been busy doing its work and research; then, when I turn up with cancer, they're there for me, ready and prepared, without request for payment. I'm in awe of what's being made available for me.

However, underneath the positive thought lies desperation: 'I'm so afraid'.

*I have emotions, but I am **not** my emotions; who am I.*

Garry and I discuss how we're getting to know the road to Nottingham, and how the best part is the journey home...with a stop at Southwell Garden Centre for well-earned scones and tea!

Actually, Nottingham City Hospital is not bad – as far as hospitals go. The modern Breast Institute building has large windows allowing sight of enclosed gardens with bamboo and other calm-inducing plants; the medical staff are attentive and compassionate, and they smile a lot! My assigned breast nurse is there to see me right through treatment. I have confidence in the departmental teams, and feel cared for...perhaps 'my' butterflies are also those felt by other patients.

Arriving at the oncology department, I try to dispel fear by finding a relaxing image: with eyes closed, I imagine *green* rising up through the floor and think about walking barefoot on lush grass.

I have a body, but I am not my body; who am I

I imagine my tummy is bathed with *orange;* the image is of a beautiful sunset which spreads below my navel, from hip to hip...even extending out beyond each side of my body.

My tummy is at the centre of my emotions. Of course it is! Whenever I feel stress, anxiety, fear, anger, my tummy squirms with tension (those butterflies) and sometimes churns with nausea, which occasionally becomes vomiting.

I have emotions, but I am not my emotions; who am I

As I sit in the waiting room, churned and scared, the image of an orange 'sunset' no longer seems fitting: the area is more like a brown and orange beach, covered with pebbles; the *brown* is the stuff of tough emotions; the pebble of anxiety is like a solid rock, tight in my gut.

I have emotions, but I am not my emotions; who am I

With focus on meditative breathing, I imagine that I can reach into my pebbles of emotions, and gently ease out the rock of anxiety; when it's free from other pebbles, I toss it away, far into the ocean, to be washed away by the tide...

Feeling calmer, I know that I ought to 'keep myself to myself': I have a habit of feeling the emotions of others, and, in the heightened atmosphere of the breast cancer waiting room, I'm likely to find myself 'sucked in' to others' pain as if it's my own...

I imagine I'm inside a colourful bubble – protected, yet oozing brightness in *pastel* shades - and as meditation takes hold, I think about filling the rooms with love; it feels good to image 'yucky' stuff being filtered away by bright light, and patients and medical staff being invigorated with *turquoise and green...*

Green persists. The oncology department floor remains bathed in green – refreshing and healing... When I'm called to the consulting room, each step feels as if my feet are on soft grass…and I imagine my doctor's direct gaze glows with *bright white*.

The images give me confidence and I'm able to listen to Dr Chan's positive words, and happily accept further information from Dr Webb: my treatment is to be part of a trial; there will be 4 lots of chemo; an intervening scan; then perhaps 4 more treatments; surgery; radiation; then injections of Herceptin. It will take a year.

I trust the doctors, and with positive steps we make our way to the next appointment: this procedure is rather like a biopsy where a marker – called a 'twirl' – is inserted in my breast; just like before, with focus on breath and breathing, it is painless; I feel brave and strong…ready for MRI.

The nurse in the MRI department warns me of the noise…

Afterwards, Garry asked, "How was that?"

"I'm not sure how people who don't meditate manage through it."

"Umm – Phil had a panic attack and had to have it stopped."

"You never said…"

"Best not to know beforehand!"

Yes! It was best not to know…that the experience of an MRI was like being Jodie Foster in the movie, *Contact*; or perhaps a character in one of Garry's Sci-fi movies being bombarded with space weapons and attacks from aliens...

Whatever I felt, whatever noise I endured, my body – and I – remained perfectly calm and still...almost into sleep...

At first I murmured, 'My dear Lord Jesus, My dear Lord Jesus...'

Then, 'I am of earth, I am of earth; I am grounded; of humus, human...'

Halfway through the 25 minute experience I thought of *purple*; I imagined bathing the MRI ring with purple, and thought: *'from now on everyone who comes through here will be bathed in purple...*

Please Angels, clear the black from here: cleanse this machine from people's fear... Fearful black becomes invigorating white; thank you.'

I felt a sense of achievement: it was 11am; I'd been through two procedures and two consultations, and felt peaceful.

I have a body, but I am not my body; who am I

I have emotions, but I am not my emotions; who am I

I have thoughts, but I am not my thoughts; who am I

The perception of colour helps to direct the process of healing; physics explains its significance: energy vibrates at different frequencies that we sense as the variety of colour and the differences of sound; a higher frequency is a more rapid vibration making a higher sound, and, through the colour spectrum, rises beyond *blues*, to the heights of *purple*.

Purple is my favourite colour.

I've begun to hate *pink:*

As this new 'journey' begins, it's challenging – without warning - to be faced with cancer charities; for example, when Garry and I tried to use shopping as an escape from our preoccupation with the disease, we found ourselves bombarded by supermarket activities promoting 'cancer awareness week': M&S were actively involved with a sponsored bike ride; and the emotional experience was much worse in Tesco where their display was made up of heart-shaped pink stickers ready to sign, 'in memory of…'

Oh, God…

Of course, there's a place for supportive, peaceful pink – it's a badge of honour for women who succeed through the wounds of breast cancer; I want to succeed too; but at the moment I have to distance myself from affirming the presence of the disease, and declare that it has no place, no value, no further purpose in me.

My colour-fuelled resolve is a determination to see my body successfully through treatment…

Comment:

'It never ceases to amaze, as well as inspire me, when the unique integrations of the spiritual with the metaphysical, the morally uplifting, the scientific, the poetic, and/or the transformational, all come pouring out of the fullness of your being – all wrapped in pink or whatever color of the day is spontaneously called forth!' Mark

11 Doing It For You

April 25th 2018

Everything I do, I do it for you:
'Look into my eyes
You will see what you mean to me
Search your heart, search your soul
When you find me then you'll search no more

Don't tell me it's not worth trying for
You can't tell me it's not worth dying for
You know it's true everything I do
I do it for you

Look into your heart
You will find there's nothing there to hide
Take me as I am, take my life
I would give it all, I would sacrifice

Don't tell me it's not worth fighting for

I can't help it, there's nothing I want more
You know it's true, everything I do
I do it for you

There's no love like your love
And no other could give me more love
There's nowhere unless you're there
All the time, all the way.' [Bryan Adams]

Dear Physical Body, you did really well yesterday;

Dear Emotions, you did really well yesterday;

Dear Subconscious Mind, Conscious Mind, Ego, you did really well yesterday.

Dear Spirit Self, you did really well yesterday.

Dear Garry, you did really well yesterday.

We stay focussed on breath, on meditative breathing, without over-excitement of our achievement.

Each part of body is acknowledged:

Beginning at my feet...

Notice toes, pads of feet, instep, heels and ankles;

Notice lower legs, calves and shins;

Notice knees, thighs, hips;

Notice spine...its base resting comfortably into the chair;

Notice tummy, abdomen, chest and breasts;

Notice shoulders, upper arms, elbows, lower arms, wrists;

Notice hands...back of hands, palms, fingers and thumbs;

Notice the gentle rise and fall of each breath...

Notice neck, chin, jaw and cheeks;

Notice eyes, nose, mouth; notice slowly swallowing...

Notice hair, scalp, forehead...the centre of forehead...

Notice the breath through nostrils...

Each inhalation...and exhalation...

With each noticing, I request that every part of my body is, **its natural self.**

My noticing affirms my love and appreciation for each part of my body;

Noticing is refreshing and invigorating;

And, at bedtime, when all parts of my body are noticed in this way, my body easily relaxes into sleep.

And so it is.

Dear Breast,

*It cannot be easy holding a 3.5 cm lump within. It's not easy knowing that a 'poisonous substance' must be used to help make you - make us - whole. But, yesterday, amidst the 'sense of injustice', you received loving care from Dr Chan. Please hold within you the memory of the moment that Dr Chan agreed with Suzanne – that you are **beautiful.** And remind yourself of how he reassuring touched our shoulder during his brief chat. My love is* *deep and strong ready for treatment to begin next Thursday, May 10th.*

Love, Suzanne

12 With Our Thought...

From the moment of waking, right through the day, fearful thoughts pierce my middle like a knife. I'm determined that every iota of unhealthy thought must leave me, my mind, and my body; this cleansing challenge will be the making – or breaking - of me...

'When the rain washes you clean, you will know, you will know...' [Fleetwood Mac]

I *know*, that in my moment of terror, my meditative mantra *worked* - dissolving the pain in my middle, and stopping tears.

I have thoughts, but I am not my thoughts; who am I

I *know*, that the frightening thought was directly felt in the centre of my body, the solar plexus.

I have thoughts, but I am not my thoughts; who am I

I *know*, that I must pay attention to my solar plexus, to 'wash myself clean' of thoughts that are unhealthy:

I have thoughts, but I am not my thoughts; who am I

As its name suggests – *solar* plexus - I imagine the middle of my abdomen is like a bright sun, shining out an ego smile.

Metaphysics suggests this is the centre of our 'mental body', the place where thoughts are processed – hence the pain in my middle when I was thinking fearful thoughts.

Solar plexus feels like the place where we receive, 'body blows'.

What must I do with 'body blows' of unhealthy thought?

My bright middle shines like the sun...but also burns like the sun.

With eyes closed and focus on meditative breathing, I imagine the 'body blow of fear' being swallowed up by my shining sun; the dark, 'sun spot' of fear is drawn into the golden yellow, where it's quickly swallowed into the glowing mass. It feels good! My 'inner sun' knows how to swiftly deal with the unhealthy matter of thoughts that are not good for me.

The image makes me smile.

I imagine a large smiley face spread across my abdomen – as though I'm wearing an 'Emoji' T shirt! My ego is happy! It knows the delight of a successful *mental transaction:*

Accept the 'thought blow', burn it with the brightest of suns, and then, from thought centre, send out a glorious smile!

Someone else may catch the smile, and will possibly have the thought: 'She's happy'! They'll feel the cosy warmth within their solar plexus, and they'll smile too.

I have thoughts, but I am not my thoughts; who am I

As I write, there's a call from Nottingham City Hospital about the next appointment – Monday April 30th at 2pm – an informative meeting for those about to receive chemo. Taking the phone call, *with calm anticipation and no pangs of anxiety*, brings confirmation of my healing mind. Indeed! Thoughts have power...a power that, once harnessed, changes the way we feel...

I have thoughts, but I am not my thoughts; who am I

Pulling clothes out of the washing machine, I find myself having a thoughtful conversation with my body:

It seems to say, *'Why do we have to do this, when left breast is at fault? Why should we be punished with chemo?'*

'No part of us is at fault. Dear body, chemo is not a punishment; you've already felt how mind, subconscious mind, emotions and ego have settled into the acceptance that chemo will help release cancer; it's not wise to think about punishment, or war;

it is wise to comfortably accept aspects of chemo that will help us, and let any parts of chemo that are not for our good flow away.'

*'So that's why we heard, **when the rain washes you clean, you will know.'***

'Exactly, dear body! You are smarter than the average body, beautiful too! We'll continue to work together to bring us back to natural wellness.'

This day began with depressive thoughts.

Winston Churchill named clinical depression, the 'black dog'...

Depressive symptoms certainly feel black.

Black is, 'what it is' because it absorbs all colour.

Absorbing all colour, absorbing everything, inclusive, knowing all...

What are you, depression?

'Darkness that helps you find Light'

Indeed. Working through depression has helped me uncover wisdom, although thinking deep thoughts can feel unpleasant. Nevertheless, I'd rather be a thinker than mindlessly plod through each day.

There's value in things that are awful...if they make you think, and feel, depth of life and living.

Before sleep last night, my thoughts were strange, unhelpful and negative; I wanted to dismiss them, have them burn into my solar plexus, and smile; but I know that each process of this journey is important; so the unusual, inner conversational thoughts need to be acknowledged:

'*Why should I, little me, think I'm important enough to have curative success?*

Why are so many people rallying round me, giving me loving support?

Why do I deserve to live beyond this?'

'*Because I want life.'*

'*You want! So what?'*

'*Because I have things to accomplish.'*

'*You think your accomplishments important?'*

'*Because of Garry.'*

'*Garry is strong; he'll be ok.'*

'*To prove it's possible.'*

'*No-one will notice, or remember.'*

It's true – people forget. I did. My school friend – also called, Suzanne; born a month before me – died of cancer 14 years ago. When her Mother phoned to tell me the news, I promised myself I'd live each day 'better', remembering Suzanne. I forgot.

I have thoughts, but I am not my thoughts; who am I

'*Father God, Earth Mother; Father God, Earth Mother'*

I slept well, after those strange thoughts.

And woke up, with more thought:

*Despite my hopes of keeping our days free of **those thoughts**, **every moment is affected by IT**. I can't do anything, or think anything, without the dull ache of thoughts about **IT**. My friends have been affected; they're sad because of **IT**. **IT'S GOT IN THE WAY. I DON'T WANT THIS. I DON'T WANT IT.***

Petulant tears, wailing tears, sorry for myself tears, angry tears, tears because of tears…are interrupted by a phone text…**reminding me of another appointment about IT.**

Deep breath. Get into the day…have a shower…

The bathroom is not a good place when I feel depressed: it's a place to have a long, private cry; depression stunts my body; I can't get into the shower. Curled up on the floor, I wail:

'Why? Why did I make this happen? Why have I ruined everything?

Even when this lump is gone, my life will be anxiety-filled, wondering if there'll be more…

'Fear the worst, hope for the best,' some stupid person told me…'

I'm disgusted by cancer in me; I'm reluctant to touch my breast…expecting the lump to be gone, and feel fear and anger that it remains…

Tears…

'Come on; think beyond the treatment. Your life is fulfilled, even if there's no creative purpose, because, **simply by being, you make the universe complete.**'

Yes! At last, tears of realisation:

'You're a lovely body; you're a lovely body; you're a lovely body...'

'When the rain washes you clean, you will know, you will know...'

'With our thought we make the world.' Buddha

13 Balance

This morning's song:

'I need more of you; changing my rain into sun;
More of you, putting my blues on the run' [Bellamy Brothers]

Yes! I need more. More inner help. More Angelic guidance. More calm concentration.

Remind myself: Thoughts and emotions settle down when there's concentration on breath, on breathing...with steady focus on the rise and fall, the rise and fall, the rise and fall...

That's all.

In some ways today is the most difficult yet – a trip to Nottingham hospital for an informative visit to the Chemo Suite.

As I emerge from the toilets in the now familiar Breast Institute, the thought returns: 'I can't believe this is happening to me, to us.'

I gulp tears away, 'This isn't real; this is not happening; it can't be…it just can't…'

The power-point presentation about the treatment and potential effects of chemo is informative, positive and sensitive; we also learn about extra provision for cancer patients – free drinks, free car park, 24/7 emergency card, a place to talk, relax and have complementary health support…

But I feel dazed, stifled, overwhelmed, confused, and very scared…

In fact, I'm terrified as I walk past the rows of patients already taking in their chemo. My brain wants to skid to a halt; my body wants me to take it far away…somewhere safe.

It's difficult to find inner calm, and challenging to follow Garry's words of advice: 'Go to your inner garden.'

I'm unable to close my eyes because I must remain alert while I'm closely surrounded in a waiting room overcrowded with patients…all happily chatting…

This can't be real…

I affirm that my 'bubble of protection' is in place, and repeat the inner affirmation: *'balanced and detached, balanced and detached…'*

After the group presentation, my individual interview

is unhurried and calm with a nurse who is positive and compassionate, but it's tough to listen to the explanation of how 'poisonous' the various concoctions are for my beautiful body, and it's plain to see that it's not easy for Garry; (later he admitted his inside knots with emotion, knowing what must be done). As the nurse talked, my eyes focus on the painting above her head – a deep purple flower.

I'm so tired, trying to rise above the 'stifling feeling', trying to grasp dates and duration of treatment, and how to monitor my body...

Please, Angels, work through this department; cleanse out the 'crud' and replace it with your Light, your Love, your Healing Power...for all who attend here...

Dear Body, I've already said, 'I'm sorry'; but, without chemo you will suffer more, and decay early. We do this together. We do this supported – by experts, and by those who love us. We do this loved by Jesus and Angels. We do this for a good reason – a reason that, at present, is unclear.

> *'Breathe through the heats of our desire*
> *Thy coolness and thy balm;*
> *Let sense be dumb, let flesh retire*
> *Breathe through the earthquake, wind and fire;*
> *Oh still small voice of calm'* [J Whittier]

It's refreshing to drive the tree-lined country roads home, to have Garry reach over to hold my hand, to notice trees laden with pink blossom, and to sit near purple thyme while we ate scones with tea...

My mind attempts to calm the ever-present emotional uncertainty:

This treatment is what is needed; it's helpful to us; people go through this bravely, successfully, every day; so, Suzanne, stop feeling sorry for yourself; stop thinking about the 'bad' and focus on the 'good'; stop wanting to wail and cry; be determined to rest now, and be thankful that the mammoth engine of the combination of many departments at Nottingham City Hospital has rolled into action for you...

And I think about the combination of medicine and metaphysics that maintains wellness:

For a body to remain healthy - to be its natural self – every system needs to flow freely;

Physically, this means:

the free-flow of blood through circulatory system,

the inward and outward flow of uninhibited breathing,

the digestive cycle of nutrients in, and excrements away,

the cleansing cycle, and elimination of toxins,

the constant regeneration of healthy cells,

the growth, and cutting back, of hair and nails,

the feminine (and masculine) cycle.

Subliminally, this means:

the flow of universal energy through the body;

the healthy flow of reciprocal giving and receiving of emotion and thought.

Wherever the flow is blocked or interrupted, there is physical disease – great or small, and 'dis-ease' of mind and spirit. Intervention is essential so that natural flow, in all areas, can resume.

My thought gives me assurance that I've done everything I can by welcoming healing intervention in every way possible:

diagnosis of the physical nature of the tumours,

use of the most appropriate forms of medication, treatments, surgery,

specific nutrients for my body; exercise; rest and sleep,

continued monitoring,

letting go of unhealthy thoughts and negative emotions which block the steady flow of mind and spirit,

healing energy to re-activate the natural flow of universal energy through every part of me.

I affirm that I am perfectly willing to accept medical treatment of chemo, surgery, radiation, medication, whilst acknowledging and thanking Healing Angels for reaching into me, transmuting the consciousness of cancer wherever and however I've been unable to heal myself.

Embracing all healing modalities, I feel immense gratitude for the skill and expertise of all who are working with me, and all who keep me and Garry in their thoughts, and I continue to ponder how to achieve healthy 'balance'.

Balance is essential for everything of the universe.

A perfect symbol of balance is the sign of *Tao* – the circle of black with white, seamlessly interlocking with an element of white within the black, and black within the white.

As I contemplated the *Tao*, I think about left as feminine, right as masculine; the feminine Yin, masculine Yang. I wonder whether black – which absorbs all colour – is feminine; and whether white – absorbing no colour – is masculine.

My thought takes me into meditation...

Noticing the rise and fall of abdomen...

*The symbol of **Tao** appears as if imprinted in the middle of my **forehead**; its circle seems to need adjustment – I imagine that I turn it, like one would slightly twist a combination dial on a bank safe...gently turning, until it makes its connection; black with white; Yin and Yang; feminine and masculine; left with right.*

I breathe, and listen to the sound of inhalation and exhalation...

*A **Tao** symbol rests in front of my **throat**; it, too, needs slight adjustment, and is turned gently, in the same way – making a connection, as one would with a combination lock; white with black; Yang and Yin; masculine and feminine; right with left.*

*The **Tao** in front of my **heart** is much larger than the previous two; its circle covers my chest; but still, it needs* adjustment, a slight turn, so that it locates perfectly; black with white; Yin and Yang; feminine and masculine; left with right.

At my **solar plexus**, there are **three Tao circles**; it seems they need to be brought together, to touch like cogs in a machine; white with black; Yang and Yin; masculine and feminine; right with left.

Two Tao circles appear in the space below my **navel**; they do not need to be brought together, simply adjusted so that they are aligned obliquely, across my tummy; their circles need turning with the same fine-tuning, as if I'm coming to the final combination of my 'safe'; black with white; Yin and Yang; feminine and masculine; left with right.

At the **base of my spine**, the **Tao** forms a sphere, like a huge gym ball, ready to practice physical balance; I imagine sitting astride the ball, tentatively lifting my feet to see if I can achieve **balance**; white with black; Yang and Yin; masculine and feminine; right with left.

Then I imagine I've entered my 'inner garden' where there's a mosaic mandala arranged on the path; I stand at the central point – a small dome, slightly raised – it's the top of the **Tao ball**! I balance on the dome, first with both feet, then eventually, standing on one foot, I perch in Yoga mudra…

With steady breathing there's **perfect balance**…and I bring myself back to full consciousness.

   '*My body was diagnosed with breast cancer, and I am healing.*'

As the day ends, Garry and I relax over coffee and gaze out over the field filled with grazing sheep; I lie back and rest my head on his stomach; then, with eyes closed, I concentrate on the rise and fall as each breath moves through my body...

Within moments it's obvious that Garry is sound asleep.

Darkness descends from my crown, through my body:

Comforting darkness;

Relaxing;

Absorbing all colour;

Absorbing love;

Absorbing everything;

Absorbing All;

Warm and expansive, like the dark night sky,

Sprinkled with dots of light;

Expansive, eternal;

Everything,

And nothing...

Each breath fills me with warm assurance; the rise and fall, the rise and fall, the rise and fall...perfectly balanced.

14 Joints

May 3rd 2018

It's strange to include a piece entitled, *Joints,* when breast cancer is the topic of these musings, but after last evening's meditation my mind suggested that *Joints* should be the positive writing of the day.

However, this morning, the emotion that reared its head for expression is *anger...*

So, before I pursue *joints, anger* must be explained...

As we prepare for the next trip to Nottingham – this time for an ECG – anger swells through me, twisting every common sense notion into negativity:

I'm angry, watching people going about their everyday business, with the assumption *they* are free from cancer...

I'm angry, thinking I'm being deceived, that people's supportive words are just an attempt to keep me feeling positive...

I'm angry when a friend says, 'Well, at least you have a date for treatment'...

Actually, I'm *infuriated*: how can having a diary entry which flags the start of chemo treatment, be *helpful?*

Perhaps Garry is right – that conversation with friends should be about *other* things;

for him, talking about each step of the medical process rakes over the pain;

for me, keeping quiet perpetuates the mistake of stuffing emotions under the proverbial carpet;

Keeping quiet feeds fear.

However, after last evening's phone call from old friends – when, once again, we revealed our 'news' - my unhappy thought returns, *'This can't be happening to me'*, followed by a night of tossing and turning...

So, there's wisdom in Garry's opinion that the topic should not be spoken of...

It will be difficult for me to keep quiet: I've always talked and talked my way through challenges.

My mind brings up today's song lyrics:

'Every time it rains, it rains pennies from heaven

Don't ya know each cloud contains pennies from heaven...

Trade them for a package of sunshine and flowers

If you want the things you love, you must have showers'

[Bing Crosby]

Having rained down my anger, I find sunshine through meditation:

Noticing each breath in…and out…

In…and out…

Joints in my body have my attention…

*I've been feeling **responsible:***

Wisdom tells me of the mistake of being responsible: being overly concerned about others; becoming too willing to help others at the expense of one's own wellbeing. Feeling responsible eventually creates an erroneous strong connection with others through the misguided notion of 'owning' them; and thereafter, 'judging' each choice they make…

Joints…

Joints grind;

they're rigid and stuck with age, and with unyielding responsibility…

Notice each knuckle of toes;

notice ankles;

Give special attention to knees;

notice hips;

notice base of spine; notice the connection of each vertebrae rising up spine, especially notice between shoulder blades, where spine curves with age and burden;

notice shoulders; elbows; wrists;

notice each knuckle in hands;

notice jaw.

Breathe…

Listen to each inhalation…and exhalation…

Breathe...

At the crown of the head, sparkles of gold appear like stars in a night sky;

Golden-ness descends, glistening into skeletal structure...

Each joint is oiled with gold: through jaw; around shoulders; into elbows, wrists and fingers; flowing from neck through every vertebrae; into hips, knees, ankles, toes...

Golden-ness throughout skeletal structure allows flowing and flexibility...

Flow with ability to respond, ability to respond, ability to respond...

An image appears of the steam infuser used in coffee shops to froth milk:

Every joint – ankles, knees, hips, base of spine, shoulder, elbows, jaw – blows out unhealthy responsibility like shots of steam, sending out the rigid grind of responsibility, judgement, resentment, frustration...

...taking in the flexible luxury of golden oil.

Meditation continues:

Entering the 'inner garden', bare feet brush against blades of grass; movement is subtle and supple...

Walking along the gravel path, fingers brush against thyme, and take in the scent...

Through the gate, walking down a sloping cliff path, onto the beach, into the ocean...

Gentle waves cover joints of feet, ankles, then knees and hips; eventually floating and drifting allows spine, shoulders, arms and head to be in the ocean blue that shimmers with golden light.

Floating...supported by gentle waves, and by the notion of Angelic hands that offer subtle direction on the tide...

Floating and flowing, blue and gold, breathing with subtle movement...the ability to respond, ability to respond, ability to respond.

Let go, let God...

Eventually back to the shallows to sit in the rippling waves... Then returning along the beach, up the cliff, through the gate into the garden, where bare feet, once more, enjoy the soft grass...

...Back to full consciousness.

No sense of being responsible – I have the ability to respond;

Ability to respond - allows me, and others, to be however we choose to be – with no sense of responsibility.

And so it is.

Love, Suzanne

15 Village Chant

May 4th 2018

Garry was enthralled to watch the function of my heart through the amazing technology of yesterday's ECG; and, as I listened to the swish of blood through the valves, I murmured, "Heart's been doing this, wonderfully, for more than 60 years!"

'There's nothing you can do that can't be done

Nothing you can sing that can't be sung

Nothing you can say, but you can learn how to play the game

It's easy

Nothing you can make that can't be made

No one you can save that can't be saved

Nothing you can do, but you can learn how to be you in time

It's easy

All you need is love

All you need is love

All you need is love, love

Love is all you need

There's nothing you can know that isn't known

Nothing you can see that isn't shown

There's nowhere you can be that isn't where you're meant to be

It's easy

All you need is love.' [Lennon and McCartney]

During today's meditation there's a mystical thought cycle:

Love of self – no matter what…

Which lets me be content in flow of universe;

Knowing self is part of flow of universe…

Allowing and acknowledging Universal Flow through me,

Is loving self – no matter what…

After our enthusiastic discussion about the incredible heart and the wonder of the human body, Garry talks more about his feelings.

He explains how it 'screws his insides', almost to tears, when he finds that I've been crying; and he doesn't enjoy reading the pieces I'm writing; it hurts him to know I'm sad inside, yet he's confident that the cancer will be cured; he expects the next few months will be difficult with the perceived challenge of encouraging me to Nottingham and supporting me through side-effects…

I tell him I'm glad to have him express his feelings, and remind him that it's rare for him to do so; our hollow laughter is laced with sarcasm - *cancer* has given us opportunity for depth of sharing…

What else has cancer achieved?

Profound realisation of life's beauty and what it really means to prepare for death and bereavement

Concentrated attention to each other, even more mutual

consideration and love

Intense attention to self-healing in all its forms

Appreciation of hospital skills

Letting go of phobia

Understanding of others in similar situations

Friends drawing close

Re-visiting former friendships

Writing

Successful meditation and deepening spirituality

Greater understanding of mind and emotions

Processing shock

Finding courage

Gaining patience

Detachment from resentment, responsibility, anger, frustration

Compassion towards others who react negatively

Letting go of ambition and undue self-expectation

Learning positive acceptance

Finding contentment in each moment - to be content 'just to be'

Satisfaction in 'being'

Walking through the village, I meet several neighbours, and as we stand in the sunshine and talk, I feel glad to have their love, their support, their willingness to listen, their encouragement and motivating comments...

It's good to talk… Isn't it?

Marching purposefully back up 'church hill', I chant:

Cancer you must go, whatever it takes, you must go; cancer you must go, whatever it takes, you must go; cancer you must go, whatever it takes, you must go…

Later, I turn to, *'A Course in Miracles'* and enjoy a meditative description:

'Beyond the body, beyond the sun and stars, past everything you see and yet somehow familiar, is an arc of golden light that stretches as you look into a great and shining circle. And all the circle fills with light before your eyes. The edges of the circle disappear, and what is in it is no longer contained at all. The light expands and covers everything, extending to infinity, forever shining and with no break or limit anywhere. Within it everything is joined in perfect continuity. Nor is it possible to imagine that anything could be outside, for there is nowhere that this light is not.' p447 [ACIM]

Comment:

'Yes, of course cancer must go. However it has stimulated some beautiful writing.' Alan

16 Dear Chemo...

May 9th 2018

Dear Chemo,

*I've struggled to refer to you as 'therapy' –
preferring to call you, Chemo-treatment! You've been 'on my mind'
for weeks, and have been a topic of conversation with me, me and
doctors, me and Garry, me and friends; but, I've not talked with you
directly.*

*You know I've resisted you; you probably remember how my
body diverted away from 'oncology' years ago at Lincoln hospital
when visiting other patients; I'd always felt sure you were not for
me.*

Definitely not for me.

*I told the breast cancer consultant you were not for me; he
lowered his eyes and muttered dubious assurance that I'd not be
forced beyond my wishes, and then mentioned mastectomy and
radiation - which would not solve my problem...at all.*

*My problem has been my stubborn resistance to you,
Chemo.*

*Thankfully, yes thankfully, I listened to Garry's wisdom,
and immediately welcomed the thought of having you help me to be
free from cancer.*

I do welcome you, Chemo.

*You too are part of the Universe; you have been wonderfully
created by clever doctors and technicians who continue to work to
make your mission better, more effective, less harmful to human
bodies.*

It's an irony that you assist wellness at the same time as making dis-ease. But, your curative mission does not have to be wholly destructive: I remember Chernobyl – how nature brings through its greenness...

*For me, with you, I desire that we work together, doing what comes naturally – you and me – that I use what is in you for my **highest good**, and that I let pass through me what is not necessary for me to assimilate.*

Let doctors and nurses, with their wisdom, oversee this healing procedure;

Let trials doctors and nurses gain knowledge so that this treatment improves conditions for others;

Let my body be conscious of its natural self;

Let cancer find its way back to its discrete place in the universe;

Let Angels oversee all this;

Let me be the perfect expression of All That Is;

And so it is.

Love, Suzanne

May 10th 2018

After another night of deep sleep, and waking without anxiety, we're up early in preparation for the drive to Nottingham City Hospital for my first treatment.

During our relaxed breakfast, Garry and I muse about an early May 10th waking 2 years ago – when we'd responded to a 2am call from our neighbour, requesting us to go to their house to sleep so they could safely leave their toddler and quickly depart to Nottingham for the birth of their second baby.

Two years on, a very different reason to be up and alert with Nottingham as the destination! Nevertheless, memories and happy photos of yesterday's early birthday cake and gifts with the now 2-year-old little girl make me smile.

Surprisingly, my mind seems to be 'smiling' too: another song presents itself in my consciousness; as I hum the tune, I feel the power of Josh Groban's voice in my head – *Un Alma Mas...*

'Ok, Universe! What's today's message within a song?'

The 'googled' translation of the lyrics thrills me:

'Un Alma Mas - One More Soul.

Don't deprive the world of love;

Without sun and rain flowers won't grow;

The miracle is in you

Don't let it die.' [Groban]

The miracle is certainly in me, plainly expressing itself as a peaceful journey to Nottingham; even when we have sight of the hospital building, I don't feel the usual lurch in my stomach; I'm amazed – *What is this calm assurance? How wonderful it feels to be free from anxiety: the hospital, for me, has turned from a place of terror into a space for healing.*

My peaceful exterior, and interior, continue as we're introduced to Claire, today's oncology nurse...

As she inserted the cannula she began to explain the detail of the day's drug concoction... With a vague smile, I shake my head, 'Please, don't tell me! It's better if I concentrate on *me;* you to do whatever needs to be done...do it around me, and let me be!'

She grinned at Garry who spontaneously became her 'nursing assistant' - following her instruction to collect a prescription from pharmacy. (We're surprised to learn that each cocktail of chemo is made individually for patients just before it is administered).

Garry's usefulness continues through the day's process: making drinks, watching my reactions, massaging feet, and creating humour for anyone prepared to listen to his quips... Without doubt, he's uncovered another skill – no wonder he's known as 'Arry, 'The General' by some friends in Evedon, and 'G-man' in Virginia Highlands, USA!

Our long day, in the research unit, is made pleasant by the natural affable personality of all nurses; they are wonderful – skilled, professional, and attentive to each patient's every need.

I try to forget drug infusion in favour of meditation, but suddenly the anxious mind, running as a constant undercurrent, makes itself known in a minor 'wobble': tears and sobs erupt...and nurses are quickly at my side:

'Is there anything we can do for you?'

'It's just...'

I wasn't sure why I'd become upset; my sudden tears are inexplicable, and so, with a shake of the head, I bring my thought and emotions under control.

In fact, I'd been perfectly calm and content while I had focus on 'me'; but as soon as my mind wandered into connection with conversations around me – of treatments, symptoms, ailments – my sensitive vulnerability is sucked into other dramas...

For a moment, I'd lost my me.

Breathe...

'Who Am I, Who Am I, Who Am I.'

Calmness returns. Thinking of blue, I gaze out of the window, 'Look, Garry, there's an aircraft high up, beyond the clouds; wonder where it's going?'

'Mr Technology' reaches for his phone to browse an app that shows details of the aircraft overhead: 'It's a 777. Flying from Brussels to New York.'

'Damn!' I laugh, 'I've missed my flight!'

Meditative thought continues:

Of a wide base chakra, exuding red;

Of the ocean, blue with rays of silver;

I feel the effects of healing energy from those thinking of me.

Later on, as I learn how to manoeuvre my drug machine attached to my very own 'dalek' contraption to the toilet, I have the thought, *'I hope the world knows how grateful I am.'*

Throughout the long procedure, and subsequent observation, our ever-cheerful nurses regularly offer us drinks and snacks.

There's a moment when I can't respond to, 'more tea?' because meditation had deepened: I felt as though I'd lost legs and arms; my body and head seemed to have disappeared; I was just heart...nothing else...nothing; my body had left me, or perhaps I had left my body... I didn't want to talk to my nurse. Why would I? I'd just found **Bliss.**

We both felt very tired as Garry drove home – knowing that we'd have to repeat the trip tomorrow, for a 10am second infusion...

Thank you:

My beautiful body; you've done well today; I am proud of you!

My glorious emotions; you've sensed goodness today; I am proud of you!

My incredible mind(s); you've thought wisdom today; I am proud of you!

My infinite spirit; you've shown us oneness today; I am proud of you!

Our supportive friends; *'your love has kept us going';* we appreciate you!

Hospital nurses, doctors, technicians...

all that *plastic* equipment... I'm grateful!

Chemo and accompanying drugs; I'm thankful for you!

'The miracle is in you
Don't let it die.'
Un Alma Mas

Love, Suzanne

Comment:

'What a strong soul you are... I hold you lovingly in my heart as you approach a week of challenges. May your body receive the chemo, may the chemo do its work, and may it leave your body much more easily... This I pray. Surrounding you with love and light, dear one!' Mar xxx

'Dear Suzanne, What a beautiful email starts my day! Thank you so much! You did wonderfully. Have another great day today and continue being your beautiful self - a shining example. The I Ching says, *"Contemplation. A great view is above. Devoted and gentle, central and correct, he is something for the world to view."* Love, Alan.'

17 Working My Way Back

May 23rd 2018

5 days in hospital

Writing has made me feel better – perhaps 'satisfied' is a better word; and I'm really glad of others' willingness to read, because another person's 'thought-filled acceptance' of each piece makes its learning 'real'.

Before receiving treatment, I'd not paid attention to information about chemo side-effects, with the idea that – if I did not 'know', maybe they would not happen.

Thankfully, Garry did the research, made practical preparation for eventualities, and gradually told me what I 'needed to know'.

You don't need to know about symptoms of side-effects! Indeed, I'd planned to avoid writing such detail; and, to be honest, the usual vocabulary of 'unwellness' does not convey the 'real feel' of the presence of chemo in the body.

For example: 'tiredness' from chemo, feels *nothing like* exhaustion, overwork, jet-lag, flu-ness, sleepiness...

In fact, there ought to be a lexicon for chemo effects - rather like Eskimos have many detailed words for 'snow'.

Since you don't need to know, why am I about to list how my body feels?

So that...

...when we meet, it will not be necessary to talk about these things...

...when you give me encouragement to be 'positive', you'll understand why I may wince and sigh...

...and...

...so that I can truthfully say, *'I'm fine.'* **F**reaked out, **I**nsecure, **N**eurotic, **E**motional. [Acronym from movie, 'The Italian Job' 2003]

So, on the twelfth day after chemo treatment, my body says to me:

Heavy head

Tight, heaviness behind eyes

Sore nose with blood spotting

Sore, burning lips

Sore, sensitive mouth

Coated teeth

Unnatural taste and smell

Jaw ache

Hoarse

Skin burn to back of hands

Fragile skin

Breathlessness, tight chest

Limbs sluggish

Legs feeling 'wooden'

Bloated tummy

Nausea

Indigestion

Bowel upset

Burning pee

Sleeplessness due to heartburn pain & irritable limbs

Tired!

My dear, beautiful body,

I'm so sorry. But, I'm so proud that you're marching bravely on. You keep telling me what you'd like to eat and drink, and we're surely doing well munching through each meal. Please be sure that chemo is not an 'infliction' upon you, but an 'accoutrement' to the real mode of healing you, healing me, healing 'us'.

Dear beautiful body; remember Chernobyl – how nature is working its way back...

'I'm working my way back to you, babe, with a burning love inside'. [The Four Seasons]

Love, Suzanne

May 24th 2018

Yesterday's writing about symptoms of 'illness' was a slight diversion from the project plan – which is about finding 'wellness'.

As I came to the end of writing *the list,* it was a delight to have my mind recall the lyrics from Frankie Valli & The Four Seasons, *'I'm working my way back to you, babe.':* My body is surely telling me that it's 'working its way' back to wellness.

Today, the main thing that stands in the way of feeling well is the dismal cycle of medication followed by side-effects.

During my recent stay in Nottingham City Hospital this problematic cycle caused the Registrar and me to draw swords: medication that he'd prescribed to stop diarrhoea, didn't; medication that was meant to prevent nausea, didn't.

When the three-times-a-day gathering of nurses over the drugs trolley took place, with conversations about what to give to whom, and what to give to whom to counter the effects of what had been given to whom... I wondered if I'd been transported to a Sci-Fi chemical establishment, being experimented upon by futuristic scientists...where patients eagerly sit up to accept their little pot of tablets, swallow, and submissively slide back between the sheets...

When I pointed out the regular pattern, of tablet – sick, tablet – tummy upset, Doctor gave me a wry smile, and shook his head dismissively, 'You're feeling sick, because you're thinking about it.'

(It only occurred to me later that he was using the mind/body connection against me, when, previously he'd dismissed such a phenomenon.)

I felt trapped.

My night-time nurse, Kim, who'd *listened* to me and suggested that a timely glass of milk, or bowl of cereal, could break the sick cycle, had gone off duty...

So, I wielded my sword... **"I want to go home."**

After further talking and listening, Doctor and I came to an understanding: it was necessary to remain in hospital because white blood cells had been wiped out. He apologised. The system of calculating chemo - using body weight and height – does not take account of metabolism. The dose for me was too strong; they'll get it right next time...(says she, cynically).

'Working my way back to you, babe,'

Body has to work its way back. Body is amazing. It works its way back, naturally.

But, how does it find its original state of perfect wellness? *How to reboot?*

For me, healing success and maintaining wellness has come about through separating the various parts of me.

I have a body, but I am not my body; who am I

I have emotions, but I am not my emotions, who am I

I have thoughts, but I am not my thoughts, who am I

I am; I am; I am

My meditative mantra eases me out of the whirl of illness panic, and brings focus back on what part of me is calm and well, and what part needs healing attention.

After thinking further about the catalogue of symptoms, and wondering whether my body will ever remember 'wellness', I recall a book by, *Richard Gerber MD, 'Vibrational Medicine for the 21st Century'*. He writes how the **blueprint** of our body, the perfect pattern of our physicality - the *etheric* body - can be seen and understood through Kirlian photography. (An experiment of this process, called the 'phantom leaf effect', shows that when a part of a leaf is amputated, photographic film shows the whole leaf intact – its etheric template remains, despite the missing piece.) I wondered if this could be why some patients who have had limbs amputated, feel irritation or pain in the area of their missing limb?

My body is working its way back. I want to help it on its journey. If my body has a **blueprint**, I want to help bring the perfect *etheric* and the suffering *physical* together, so that they merge back to total wellness:

With eyes closed, I find myself in my inner garden; my bare feet luxuriate on the soft grass, a warm breeze wafts against my skin, I turn my face up to the blue sky.

Mindfully, I walk along a gravel path; each step is like a warm massage to the soles of my feet.

I make my way along the lavender border, to a gate at the end of the garden.

Through the gate, I find myself at the top of a cliff, and stand for a while, enjoying the ocean, the horizon, the expanse of blue sky.

Gradually, I make my way down a sloping path to the beach; my toes enjoy the grains of warm sand; I stoop to grab a handful and as I allow the sand to pour through my fingers I recall the profound verse:

'To see a world in a grain of sand

And a heaven in a wild flower

Hold infinity in the palm of your hand

And eternity in an hour.' [William Blake]

As I walk the beach, I become aware of each aspect of 'who I am':

I am **a large bubble** that moves easily over the sand; translucent and many coloured, I glisten in the sunshine…

I look down as my bubble parts at my feet, easing itself up over my head, to hover over my body; I realise it's my **Spirit**, always around me…

As I begin to stroll towards the ocean, I notice someone has hold of my hand… And, as I look to my right, there's a string of me, like sisters, holding hands, making our way together to the rippling waves…

It feels like a girls' beach party: with spirit bubble overhead, the various parts of me separate - my **physical** body, my **emotional** self, my **mind** and **subconscious mind**…and **ego has** to be there!

Then I feel little fingers clutch my left hand; I look down at a little girl, about 8 years old, I know her as my **'inner child'**.

I squeeze her hand, and she smiles, 'I like the seaside!'

'I know you do, Suzy; you're my brave Little One.'

We stand in a row, enjoying the waves breaking over our knees, until one by one, each part breaks handhold to float separately

94

in the shallows. My inner child and I watch as the bubble spreads over the other parts of me, like a blanket over the sea, a purple haze over blue...

'They're bathing, aren't they?'

'They are. Bathed and being cleansed with Love.'

My inner child wanders to play and splash in the sea; I notice how all blue that I've been seeing – of ocean and sky - is now a deep penetrating blue...from somewhere distant, yet ever close: blue above me, around me, underneath, and completely suffused through me; I feel lifted up, and floating...

I focus on breath and breathing, allowing, accepting, acknowledging...

Gradually I float above the ocean; eyes closed, I am a floating sandwich: sea...sea with parts of me...blue...me...blue...purple bubble...sky.

I can stay like this forever...

But then, blue's activity seems to be complete; as I float, other parts of me rise up from the ocean to join me – subconscious mind, mind, emotion, ego – assimilating back into my whole.

'New every morning is the love

Our wakening and uprising prove;

Through sleep and darkness safely brought

Restored to life and power and thought.' [John Keble]

I'm back on the warm sand. The bubble is no longer overhead: I know that it - my spirit - has resumed its place, totally surrounding me in everlasting loving protection.

I smile at the little girl, now busy making sandcastles; and as I begin to walk up the beach, she runs after me, 'Are we going back to the garden now?'

'We are; I'll rest there for a while; perhaps have a sleep; I know I'm going to feel even better.'

'Do I have a blueprint too?'

'You do, Little one; in fact, your blueprint is exactly like mine!'

Comment:

'Dear cynical Suzanne,

Congratulations on being home again and waking in your old liveliness, after a good night's sleep. I hope today is a good day and that you will be able to manage with a less near-lethal dose of the chemo next time. Your body sure has a lot to say. But is hasn't said "no" to further chemo, so please give it my congratulations for courage.

I asked the I Ching if there was anything further to say, and it gave big encouragement. Here is the essence of it: *"It furthers one to undertake something for that is devotion to the command of heaven."* That's it! Keep going!' Love, Alan

'Suz...again I am deeply moved by the bare and honest truth of your sharing and description of what you are going through...if one has not experienced the awful side effects of chemo, it is difficult to understand...however, your descriptions help. Am appreciating how lovingly you address your body and even the chemo. Hope each day you feel better. Love you,' Mar

18 Follow You, Follow Me

May 25th 2018

In a previous piece, I listed what cancer has achieved. Top of the list has to be: *The realisation of the beauty of life, and what it really means to prepare for death/bereavement.*

Now, two weeks after the first chemo treatment, my thoughts turn to what that experience has taught me:

First, and most surprising: the calm acceptance of the cannula in the back of my hand, and a composed allowing of the substance into my vein. During the two hour procedure, I remember sitting back, thinking about the country-road journey to the hospital, of lilac and wisteria; and as I looked out at the bird deterrent spikes on the hospital roof, I imagined each spike topped with pink hearts – like those scattered through texts from my encouraging friends.

Then, a new understanding of how to care for my body: Through years of early morning psychosomatic vomiting, I learned to abandon food until coffee time, and then gorge chocolate. Whenever I caught normal stomach bugs, I knew to sip water until my tummy was ready for dry toast and tea.

These sicknesses were a *response to fear*, and the *result of infection*.

Chemo sickness is *reaction to an invasion*.

Even now, 14 days later, my body feels weakened by

toilet trips several times a day, but, so different from the other maladies, I feel somehow physically lively, although I have doubts about my sprightliness when I see the pale face in the mirror.

And - totally different from the other types of stomach upset - my body demands frequent food: carrots, and more carrots; milk, and more milk; oat cereal; green tea; yogurt; macaroni cheese; beef burger and chips! *Keep feeding me! Keep feeding me stodge rather than food that's healthy!*

And, chemo treatment has brought new learning about *relationships* – particularly my most precious relationship: me with Garry.

I've heard about couples splitting up after having worked through cancer, and never understood how that could possibly happen. However, after the first chemo, when my body reacted with unimaginable pain and discomfort, our 38 years of consistent mutual friendship and happiness showed a few slight cracks...

We'd been used to controlling our lives, planning and doing things together; we'd always decided on a combined direction...

This strong togetherness had brought us through the initial shock of cancer diagnosis...

Garry had taken control of the plan – certain that he knew what to do to bring comfort; he'd done research, and *made sure* he'd got whatever was necessary for me...whatever...the utmost...

Then, my body showed unexpected weakness, and I crumbled.

This was not part of the plan.

He did not know what to do.

He did not know what to do.

He felt failure.

Fear.

Anger.

Anger expressed by slamming the door.

In the hollow silence I remembered his initial expression of misery, 'Suppose now I'll have to learn to use the washing machine.'

I wanted to scream, '*You* said I should accept chemo!'

Our tentative attempt at argument resolution was a perfunctory coming together: he set a cup of tea beside me, and left me to drink it alone.

Was this how it was going to be?

If so, I'd rather die.

We brought ourselves round, separately, by solitary thinking:

For me, having dissected the incident, I realised being alone with a cup of tea was not a state of disagreement and anger - it was normal behaviour! We'd always disappeared into our own little worlds (me to write and meditate, him to watch TV) then re-emerge after a while to pursue projects together.

For him, he used the solitude to construct another plan: more ideas to make everything right for me – a new movie that we could watch together; a trip to M&S food to fill the freezer full of easy dishes…

He resumed his sturdy determination to make sure I was totally taken care of.

He's my rock.

He's dependable.

I couldn't have got this far without him.

He couldn't have got this far without me.

'Follow you, follow me' [Genesis] has been 'our' song from the moment of our engagement; his expressed sentiment to me:

'Stay with me,

My love I hope you'll always be

Right here by my side if ever I need you

Oh my love

In your arms

I feel so safe and so secure

Every day is such a perfect day to spend

Alone with you

I will follow you, will you follow me

All the days and nights that we know will be

I will stay with you, will you stay with me

Just one single tear in each passing year

With the dark

Oh I see so very clearly now

All my fears are drifting by me so slowly now

Fading away

I can say

The night is long but you are here

Close at hand, oh I'm better for the smile you give

And while I live

I will follow you, will you follow me

All the days and nights that we know will be

I will stay with you, will you stay with me

Just one single tear in each passing year there will be.' [Genesis]

Comment:

'THANKS, SUZANNE. HE'S NO ORDINARY ROCK - THE SORT THAT CROWNS ARE MADE OF. YOU CHOSE WELL. KEEP GOING, BOTH OF YOU.' X ALAN

19 Mamma Mia

Holiday Sunday May 27th 2018

I'd not expected to be writing today, but a 2am wakeup gives me more to share.

The early hours' nausea and tummy upset brings concern:

Have I been expecting too much? Hoping for physical 'normality' too soon?

Temperature - a consistent 36.6.

Perhaps the nausea is a symptom of anxiety. Tuesday looms - another appointment with Dr Chan, and then Friday…treatment number 2…

Yes, there's anxiety. I'd asked whether to expect a similar reaction with the next chemo - I'd heard that reactive symptoms become worse with successive treatments…

As I write, I want to cry…

Doctor had assured me the reaction would not be as bad: they'd got it wrong the first time; he said if they got it wrong again, they were not doing their job.

Yes, I must cry…

Wisdom takes over:

Milk. Get some milk.

You know these symptoms; they come in waves, indicating that there's a residue of 'stuff' that needs to be cleansed away.

I sip milk and meditatively watch my breath…

Closing my eyes, my mind guides me to the inner garden:

Once there, I make my way to the fountain; standing under the sparkling water, I welcome the tumbling spray over and into my body; it feels as though the stream of cleansing and refreshment enters my spine; the flow descends through and around every vertebrae, searching out every minute speck of chemo that doesn't need to be there...washing and clearing, cleansing and healing...

Yes, please find every speck; please wash through my body; make sure all that is not for my good is taken away with the flow, out to the ground, out through the ground, back into Earth Mother to be taken unto herself for transmutation – for Her to do what She does, naturally...like Chernobyl...

Please help me let go of thoughts and feelings that get in my way...

Let go, let God; let go, let God; let go, let God

Breathe...

Remember Who I Am; I Am, I Am, I Am...

Eventually I wake again at 9.15am!

'Child of mine, child of mine

Oh yes, sweet darling, so glad you are a child of mine.' [Carole King]

My Dear Lord Jesus,

Thank you that I am your child, your loving child, who wants to love, and be loved...just because I got up this morning.

Love, Suzanne

May 30th 2018

Everyone is delighted after yesterday's appointment with Dr Chan, where his measurement of the 'lump' showed its size to have decreased from 4.5x3.5cm to 2.5x2.5cm.

I didn't ought to be anxious: treatment 2 is expected to be easier because chemo dose has been reduced by 20% and I've been laden with more medication to prevent sickness and acid reflux and this...and that...

As I write, my shorn hair falls on to the keyboard; I'm like a moulting squirrel!

Contemplation takes me back to the inner garden; this time, to the *tree:*

The tree is ancient; its girth enormous, its bark deeply indented with rough crevices; its gnarled roots twist over the ground.

I want to show my love for the tree, just as I feel it loves me.

As I flatten my chest against its trunk, and attempt to wrap my arms around it, I feel the pulse of its life-force - the same life-force that channels through me.

For a long time, I've wanted to be a channel – a channel of peace and wisdom...

'I have a dream...' [Abba]

I didn't have such dreams when I was a little girl; I always wanted to be a teacher, even though each morning's journey to school was fraught with anxiety: as I walked from home, across a field towards the bus stop, I used to pause every few steps to turn and wave to my Mum.

Another song, from, '*Mamma Mia*', reminds me of those mornings:

> '*Schoolbag in hand, she leaves home in the early morning*
>
> *Waving goodbye with an absent-minded smile;*
>
> *I watch her go with a surge of that well-known sadness*
>
> *And I have to sit down for a while*
>
> *The feeling that I'm losing her forever*
>
> *And without really entering her world*
>
> *I'm glad whenever I can share her laughter*
>
> *That funny little girl.*
>
> *Slipping through my fingers all the time*
>
> *I try to capture every minute*
>
> *The feeling in it*
>
> *Slipping through my fingers all the time.*
>
> *Do I really see what's in her mind*
>
> *Each time I think I'm close to knowing*
>
> *She keeps on growing*
>
> *Slipping through my fingers all the time.*' [Abba]

My Mother struggled to understand me, just as I struggle to understand myself! Her comments varied, from bewilderment: 'You are funny,' to frustration: 'Be a good girl, do the right thing,' and often: 'I wish I was you, Suzanne.'

I don't think she'd 'wish she was me' right now…

However, she gifted me the utmost privilege: allowing me to be present, holding her hand, as she passed away. That precious moment, with Garry sitting close by, confirmed for me that, *'I believe in Angels.'* [Abba]

As my garden meditation continues - *standing by the tree – I'm not surprised to be greeted by Angels and Spirit Guides. I'm invited to sit with them in a circle of ornate chairs – unusual for a garden gathering!*

I rest my hands on the elaborate chair arms, close my eyes, and focus on my breath. The occasion is important, but I feel comfortable and at ease.

I know there's 'conversation' around the circle, yet I hear no words...

Words cannot express what is being communicated; neither can thoughts or feelings interpret the message...

I breathe...

And just know...

Suddenly, I want to cry: 'Please, please, show me what I need to know; help me to be, how I ought to be; please let me not waste this moment. Please, show me how **to do the right thing.'**

The circle of chairs is gone. I press my face against the tree, and feel its warmth. Maybe I said the 'wrong' thing? Perhaps my desperation spoiled the moment? Frustration at my stupidity melts as my mind hears the song:

'I have a dream, a song to sing

To help me cope with anything

If you see the wonder of a fairy tale

You can take the future even if you fail

I believe in angels

Something good in everything I see

I believe in angels

When I know the time is right for me

I'll cross the stream – I have a dream

I have a dream, a fantasy

To help me through reality

And my destination makes it worth the while

Pushing through the darkness still another mile

I believe in angels

Something good in everything I see

I believe in angels

When I know the time us right for me

I'll cross the stream – I have a dream.' [Abba]

There are no words to express how I feel: that the dream is becoming reality, for me, through me.

Comment:

'We're both really pleased to read that the lump has diminished! Well done.'

'That's beautiful, Suzanne. I know that you have the ability to bring dreams to reality.' Love, Alan

'Dearest Suzanne, Hope you have a good sleep and that you feel rested and ready for tomorrow's treatment. As always, we send lots of luck and love and hope that your sensitivity is correctly taken into account!!!! Goodnight to you both.' Xxxxxxx

20 Then And Now

June 13th 2018

For several days, a 1965 song by the Kinks has been playing through my mind:

'I'm so tired

Tired of waiting

Tired of waiting for you.' [Kinks]

The lyrics are hardly appropriate:

With Garry always anticipating my every need – I'm not tired of waiting;

With friends constantly enquiring, giving loving support – I'm not tired of waiting;

With neighbours turning up with meals, shopping, and helping with chores – I'm not tired of waiting...

Incidentally, Jane Fonda, in this month's *Vogue*, was asked:

What's the key to being a good friend?

Her response: *'Being constructively honest, showing up fully, giving encouragement and care.'*

Thank you, my friends!

Maybe I was 'tired of waiting' on June 1st – the date of second chemo treatment?

We'd both felt anxious, waking at 3am; but by 7am I'd found a state of 'readiness-for-anything'. As we walked towards the hospital building, we both felt cheerfully relieved that we'd arrived, and glad that the waiting area for oncology day-treatment was not crowded, as I'd feared. But then, after several attempts to insert a cannula - my body was definitely resisting intervention – I *was* 'tired of waiting'.

And, after a further 2 hour wait for my chemo prescription to arrive, we were *definitely* 'tired of waiting'.

Then, towards the end of the treatment, a sudden intolerance to the final drug meant that an anti-inflammatory infusion had to be introduced before resuming chemo at half flow rate.

So, after 7 hours 'hooked up', I was *undoubtedly*, 'tired of waiting'.

In the days following this second treatment, I learn to use a new phrase:

That was then, this is now

That was then, this is now:

Whenever I feel that discomfort is intolerable...

'That was then, this is now'

...the discomfort is not as bad as a moment ago

When my body feels inert...

'That was then, this is now'

...movement has improved from 5 minutes ago

When I feel out of touch with my body, with little idea of how to manage its needs...

'That was then, this is now'

...another breath towards my body making its way back

When, a week after treatment, my thought plummets the depths: *'God has deserted me'*...

'That was then, this is now'

...that moment's thought was then; this now, is an Holy Instant

Whenever I think about what I might be able to do soon...

'That is then, this is now'

...my thought lets go of impatience, and settles into the moment of now

Eventually, I notice how my body can cuddle into the duvet, feeling snuggly and sleepy, rather than tense and inert; and how walking resumes its natural way, rather than wooden and determined.

That was then, this is now

Throughout days of physical struggle, I've seemingly been unable, unwilling, to use meditative techniques; instead, my imaginal mind takes me for frequent strolls to places I've known and loved – through parks, around lakes, throughout interesting neighbourhoods – and I feel the benefit of thinking of blue sky, greenery and sunshine.

'Focus on anything that gives you peace.

This will pass.

Keep on walking.' [Mar]

Unfortunately, I lost my Way.

Overwhelmed by physical challenges, my thought has only been about chemo treatment and symptoms, with little notion of healing.

I lost the focus upon cancer, and of the essential need to keep on, keeping on, letting go of its presence within and around my being.

Keep on walking.

'I'll walk in the rain by your side
I'll cling to the warmth of your hand
I'll do anything to keep you satisfied
I'll love you more than anybody can
And the wind will whisper your name to me
Little birds will sing along in time
Leaves will bow down when you walk by
And morning bells will chime
I'll be there when you're feeling down
To kiss away the fears if you cry
I'll share with you all the happiness I've found
A reflection of the love in your eyes
And I'll sing you the songs of the rainbow
A whisper of the joy that is mine
And leaves will bow down when you walk by
And morning bells will chime
I'll walk in the rain by your side
I'll cling to the warmth of your tiny hand
I'll do anything to help you understand
And I'll love you more than anybody can' [Denver]

Comment:

'My Dear Suzanne, Your writing is so beautiful, honest, and conveys so deeply what you are experiencing. Please don't judge

112

yourself for occasionally straying from your deepest knowing…you are simply experiencing that which is so difficult…be gentle as you experience it all…I love you. Your writing is so poignant…helps me to understand what you are going through. And makes me feel close to you.' Mar.

21 Thousandfold

June 18th 2018

It's a week since we visited Nottingham City Hospital for a second ECG – checking that Heart is maintaining its Natural Way through chemo treatment.

The week has been peace-filled, without medication, without the *need* for medication.

There are no words to express the wonder and gratitude at the amazing way the human body steadily, sturdily and incredibly finds its way back to its Natural Way of Being.

I am in awe.

Thank you, My Dear Body, for working your way back to near normalcy; thank you that you will continue your self-healing process until you have recovered your normal balance; thank you that you have accepted the presence of chemo, helping every aspect of us to affirm that cancer no longer has a place within and around our being; thank you that you are preparing yourself, and are willing to accept further treatment according to the wisdom of doctors. Dear Body, I love you; it is a privilege to live within you.

Indeed, *privilege* was the word that floated through my mind as I relaxed during the Electrocardiogram procedure:

The privilege of having doctors request that my heart should be monitored by an amazing machine;

the privilege of being able to see heart working, and hear the wonderful sound of vitalising blood pumping through its cavities.

'How comforting,' I thought, 'for babies to have such a sound as they prepare for the world... My heart's been steadily beating, almost unnoticed.'

Actually, Heart, like the rest of my body, *has* been noticed - through meditative practice and during my daily shower where I habitually talk to body, appreciating the wonder of its natural function.

However, in the week following chemo treatment 2, I struggled to find the wherewithal for my everyday spiritual practice; all I seemed able to do was to lie and allow everything to take its natural course...

SHOCK was the perfect word to describe my situation.

Shock quietened my emotions;

Shock stilled my mind;

Shock took me to a deep spiritual place, called 'Ting – The Cauldron'; a place which I think of as 'the womb of God'; a place where all that I could sense was the *Heartbeat of God*.

The thought and prayers of those caring about us helped me through that dark week, and enabled me to emerge...towards wellness and into peace.

I feel *privileged* to have had this experience; for having been through it, I am changed: *'Shock brings success'.* The success for me is *clarity: that the presence of cancer has not only shown me how to let go of anger, resentment, responsibility, and feeling indignant, but also it has freed my heart space, so that any sense of distance between ego and spirit evaporates, and I know - I AM.*

As this wealth of learning seats into my being and suffuses my consciousness, there can be no turning back; wisdom has brought *clarity,* and is showing me the value of *authenticity* and *integrity,* which brings *inspiration.*

Meditation continues to show me The Way:

This image is called, 'Thousandfold'...

With eyes closed, I focus on breath, on breathing;

At the centre of my Heart there appears a small, bright green dot;

With each breath, I watch the dot and appreciate the freshness of its green;

It feels like new life, of spring, of vibrancy and youthful energy;

It is my Heart's jewel.

It grows with each breath;

Now, like a flower, new petals emerge from its centre;

Each lime green petal is closely squeezed against its neighbour –

My Heart flower is like the pom-pom species of dahlia.

As each petal comes forth, it brings with it 'stuff' that seems unheartlike:

Indeed, Heart, like an auger, brings forth detrimental thought, unhealthy emotion…

Spewing each out while unfolding further green goodness.

This is Heart's ease – its way of being: it loves to cleanse and heal;

With each unfold and outreach, it expands,

growing stronger, larger, more vibrant, more receptive:

*It unfolds **thousandfold**.*

My breath focus continues;

Flower of vibrant green spreads across my chest;

It extends to my breasts, and over my abdomen;

Each breath feeds its beauty, its love,

Its passion, its compassion.

I am all Heart;

And upon receiving my invitation, Spirit becomes my All.

I AM.

And so it is.

I feel privileged to see and recount such images, and privileged too to have a wealth of others' creativity flow through my mind, to be able to use lyrics as a perfect expression of the present moment:

Today's gift: *'Hold on tight to your dream.'* [Electric Light Orchestra]

And this:

'A flower has opened in my heart...

What flower is this, what Flower of spring,

What simple, secret thing?

It is the peace that shines apart,

The peace of daybreak skies that bring

Clear song and wild swift wing.

Heart's miracle of inward light,

What powers unknown have sown your seed

And your perfection freed?...

O flower within me wondrous white,

I know you only as my need

And my unsealed sight.' [Sassoon]

Love, Suzanne

Comment:

'Thank you, Suzanne. *"Nothing transforms things so much as the Ting. It means taking up the new. Through gentleness the ear and eye become sharp and clear."* With much love, Alan. PS, *"A flower has opened"* is one of my favourites.'

22 C6

June 20th 2018

⸱ It's Wednesday. As I count each 'good' day down to Friday – the date of chemo treatment 3 – I feel afraid.

My mind tries to analyse why, after yesterday's meeting with Dr Chan's Registrar, I had to cry; there was no reason for tears: the doctor was pleased that my body was tolerating chemo well, and suggested that the cancer lump had diminished by a further 0.5 cm.

'Is that *all?*' I thought. I'd hoped there'd be a bigger reduction in size, like the last time...

My pessimistic personality grasped for further positives... He *was* positive... But my mind is invaded by anxious thoughts:

'They're deliberately talking up the situation; everyone does; everyone keeps telling me to be strong, to be positive... it's hard to trust what people say...'

The research nurse's information about another MRI after the 4th treatment, and perhaps another biopsy, crowds my mind; my thought insists on finding potential problems: a biopsy means they're not sure...maybe there'll still be cancer present after treatment 4. What then? Must I have another four treatments after all?

I thought I'd been working so hard to heal.

But really, not hard enough.

I continue to struggle with thoughts and feelings that are not conducive to healing cancer:

My waking thought is about man's inhumanity to man.

*Each 'good' day, when I venture outside, I feel **inferior**, afraid of what neighbours may think about me wearing a hat; they're sure to have guessed the truth of my disguised baldness... I feel dismayed at the blemishes on my face...*

*I feel **ashamed at having cancer.***

I allow feelings of misery about our life being dominated by cancer and chemo.

Periodically the thought returns: 'I can't believe this is happening to me.'

And I wonder where the experience is leading...

*I'm not afraid of dying. I know that the process of leaving one's body is blissful and light-filled. But I do not wish to make this transition until my life, this time, is **fulfilled**. **I have to make the experience of having had cancer in my body worthwhile.***

I have a body, but I am not my body.

I have emotions, but I am not my emotions.

I have thoughts, but I am not my thoughts.

Who Am I

Who Am I

Who Am I

For a while, I've wanted to write a piece entitled, 'C6'.

C6 is the design name of unusual jewellery by Anne Cohen that Garry and I came across in Stavanger, Norway; there, we purchased a ring, and later - for my 60th birthday - Garry gave me a matching bracelet; the contemporary pieces are black with one tiny diamond; the light-weight, simple beauty makes me think of a bright little star against a dark sky.

C6 – Carbon

Carbon; the elemental 'stuff' of the universe.

Carbon...graphite...

Carbon...diamond...

Carbon...my body...

Who Am I

Who Am I

Who Am I

From Anne Cohen's website: 'The design concept of C6 is shaped by the uniqueness and duplicity of the element it is named after and with the concept carrying the chemical name for carbon in the periodic table. The C6 is based on usage of pure carbon atoms materialised in multiple forms, with the jewellery composed of carbon in two completely different appearances – namely graphite and diamond. Combining science *and aesthetics, the C6 design concept brings the diamond back into a beautiful cradle of its natural element.*

The element C6 is the basis for our living world. It is found deep inside our planet, in living creatures, in the air that we breathe, and throughout the universe. Without C6 there would be no life. Created by supernova stardust, C6 spread into the universe and formed the planets and life on earth. Graphite and diamonds – the two materials constituting the C6 concept – are allotropes of carbon, pure forms of the same element that differ in structure.

The C6 design concept is based on the philosophy of C6 as a symbol of life. Black as coal and clear as light. This duplicity and the elements' duality embody the magic of the elemental cornerstone, C6 of the living world. The design also plays with time, space and being. An evolution from supernova explosions to modern technology. An existential state of mind by the simplicity of C6 and yet complex.' [Anne Cohen]

Who Am I

Who Am I

Who Am I

Playing with time, space and being.

I have a wonderful carbon-based body, the stuff of the Universe.

My body's stuff of the Universe has gone awry, duplicating itself in a mistaken way – called cancer.

My body and I have welcomed stuff of the Universe, called chemo, to arrest the activity of cancer.

The 'black' integrates with 'white' creating 'beauty';
the All of the Universe working together.

Who Am I

Who Am I

Who Am I

I have a body; a beautiful, amazing body; but I am not
my body.

I have emotions; emotions that bring tears; but I am
not my emotions.

I have thoughts; thoughts that can be destructive; but I
am not my thoughts.

Who Am I

I have a wonderful carbon-based body that has
seamlessly integrated my emotions and thoughts, and is
miraculously imbued with Spirit... My Spirit... The Spirit that
permeates The Multiverse from Infinity, as The Infinite...

Oh God, Who Am I, Who Am I, Who Am I

'Some days are diamonds, some days are stones

Sometimes the hard times, won't leave me alone

Sometimes a cold wind blows a chill in my bones

Some days are diamonds, some days are stones

Now the face that I see in my mirror

More and more is a stranger to me

More and more I can see there's a danger

In becoming what I never thought I'd be.' [Denver]

Breathe… Come on, Suzanne, breathe;

Watch the Thousandfold flower infinitely unfolding your heart…

Breathe…

Blue sky for a new day…

Time for today's plan – to go out for a drive…

I can't believe this has happened to me

The normal doesn't seem normal anymore

The wonder of the Universe seems somehow closer…and yet farther away

A star, shining a long time ago, in the dark sky…

Comment:

'Dear Suzanne, thank you for sharing your thoughts. Blue sky for a new day, bright star for a new life. Your life. What an adventure! My love is with you,' Alan

23 Toes In Dust

June 21st 2018

What a difference a day makes! After yesterday's worries, fears and tears, today a feeling of physical, emotional and mental normality. Thank you!

I feel well-prepared for the third chemo treatment, tomorrow, and keen to move away from physical symptom side-effects; so my repeated word of the day is simply,

'Healing'... with accompanying thought of colours of green/turquoise/aqua.

Healing, healing, healing...

Healing for me, for you, for others, for the world – it's all the same.

Last night I slept on silk!! I'd been browsing varieties of bed linen, hoping to find something that would be rejuvenating, especially as, once again, over the next few days, I'm likely to be spending extra time in bed. Retail staff in John Lewis bedding department were helpful; following their advice, I came home with 'soft and silky' duvet cover and sheet in cool ice blue, and was easily persuaded to purchase extra luxury with a pure silk pillowcase...my bald head feels cradled in luxurious comfort!

Actually, meditation has led me from head to the other end of my body – to *toes*...

...with a new meditative image:

Breathing gently, mindfully, attention is upon toes;

I am bare-foot on dusty ground;

I ought to be gazing at the road ahead,

Or making a decision to take a new path...

Instead, I watch toes flex in the hot dust.

My next step has to be mindful:

I watch as heel, side of foot, ball of foot, then toes

Flatten against the dust.

Foot remains stationary as toes feel and clench into the dirt.

I wait, and make ready for next step.

The other foot copies its sister:

Heel, side of foot, ball of foot, then toes

Flatten against the dust.

This foot also remains stationary for the same procedure -

Of toes flexing and clenching into the dirt.

The mindful exercise continues…

I have no idea whether I am on the 'right' road;

No thought about my journey;

No sense of my destination;

Just attention on toes, attentiveness to each step…

After a while, my toes show me their value, their unique ability:

Lingering on one step, toes adjust themselves very slightly;

I feel the adjustment in the base of my spine –

A sense of opening, of receptiveness

that sends energy up through vertebrae…

to the 'small' of my back;

Another slight toe movement -

A slight clench of toes against the dust;

The adjustment now takes place higher up, between shoulder blades…

THIS is where the healing unfolds:

A gentle spinal adjustment from shoulder blades,

Up to neck;

Supporting and relaxing the base of head;

Uplifting...

Support and upliftment draws back the skin of my face,

Gently stretching back eyebrows and eyes,

Easing back against temples;

Stretching forehead, opening Third Eye...

My spine, my back, feels adjusted, uplifted;

I am taller;

Chest and breast expand,

Inflating lungs,

Causing deep inhalation...

And exhalation;

My closed eyes feel wide open,

Nasal avenues clear,

Forehead lines are smoothed away,

Jaw relaxes into a slight smile.

Toes have affected my body from toe to top;

I'm ready for another step.

This time my footfall is lighter, slighter,

Although toes still adjust into the dust,

Rippling healing energy through my body.

'Tiny toes, your minute action

Has magnificent effect.

Thank you!'

I believe that such delightful images come to me because of the joy of teaching young children; my carefully stepping toes remind me of hearing them sing:

'One more step along the world I go

From the old things to the new

Keep me travelling along with you.

Round the corner of the world I turn

More and more about the world I learn

And the new things that I see

You'll be looking at along with me.

As I travel through the bad and good,

Keep me travelling the way I should

Where I see no way to go

You'll be telling me the way I know.

And it's from the old I travel to the new,

Keep me travelling along with you.

Give me courage when the world is rough

Keep me loving though the world is tough

Leap and sing in all I do

Keep me travelling along with you.

You are older than the world can be

You are younger than the life in me

Ever old and ever new

Keep me travelling along with you.' [Carter]

Yes! To 'leap and sing' in all I do...

Indeed, someone has commented on the variety of music that appears in each writing; I've decided that, *'God gave rock and roll to you, gave rock and roll to you; put it in the soul of everyone.'* [Kiss] is an ideal way to start tomorrow!

God gave rock and roll to me!

Love, Suzanne x

Comment:

With a fulfilled sense of well-being, I hear words from those now in spirit:

'God bless you, and your work,' Enid.

'Amen,' Ethel.

24 The Blip

June 23rd 2018

Yesterday, the date of my third chemo treatment, was a very good day: a peaceful drive to Nottingham; vein accepted the cannula *first* time; my body easily accepted the drugs, having an addition of antihistamine and steroids to accompany a slower rate of infusion for the final drug – docetaxel – that body resisted during 2nd treatment.

As Garry and I snacked our way through the day, nurse Amy told us of her Mother's cancer diagnosis some years ago, how they thought of the disease as a *blip* to be treated and moved through; she explained how the experience had drawn her family closer together, changed their attitude to life and living – taking opportunities without procrastination. I found her philosophy most refreshing; she thought meditation was a good idea.

Treatment lasted from 12 til 5pm. During that time my mind repeated one precious word: *healing, healing, healing.*

In my inner garden, I walked barefoot on luscious grass; and then found myself lying stretched out, relaxed and comfortable; spreading my arms into the blades of grass, it felt as though green seeped through my body... Then I sensed healing hands gently pressing against the back of my head, supportive, lifting head, neck and shoulders... My head filled with turquoise, green made its way to Thousandfold at my heart.

Thousandfold, like a dahlia, continued to unfold from Heart Chakra whilst I noticed another flower – a water lily across my abdomen...

Lily.

'Suzanne' means 'Lily'.

Water lilies have slender, strong roots that delve deep into depths, finding stability and nutrients; their leaf pads achieve balance on water's surface; their flowers unfurl pink and white petals in beautiful stillness...

'Each Lily of Forgiveness offers all the world the silent miracle of love.' [A Course in Miracles.]

After treatment, Garry and I enjoyed the drive home where I was glad of a cleansing shower, while he prepared our tasty dinner.

We ate outside in our newly erected garden 'pod' – a futuristic spherical garden room that gives protection from cool winds and direct sunlight, allowing us to enjoy the view of the fields beyond our home; the decision to have this 'out-of-house' freedom is a direct result of having had cancer!

As Garry and I watched the sun set, he squeezed my toes and murmured, *'You're a good girl.'*

We both felt grateful for a very good day.

Moving into another day, after a sleep filled night, body aches from eyelids downwards; walking to bathroom feels wooden, with each step seeming to need direction...

While I ate Garry-made porridge, my mind was encouraged by the lyrics of another song:

> *'Every breath you take*
>
> *Every move you make*
>
> *Every step you take*
>
> *I'll be watching you.*
>
> *Every single day*
>
> *Every word you say*
>
> *Every game you play*
>
> *Every night you stay*
>
> *I'll be watching you*
>
> *Oh can't you see*
>
> *You belong to me.'* [The Police]

Healing, healing, healing...

Green and turquoise...

Comment:

'What a great ending to Session Three. Well done, Suzanne.'
Love, Alan

25 Billions And Billions

June 27th 2018

It seems that after chemo treatment on a Friday, the
worst days are Monday and Tuesday; the change into
Wednesday is remarkable – well-done, body!

That having been said, this time's side-effects were
nothing compared to treatment 1 and 2 – just feeling
physically flushed and 'wooden'; and, apart from seven daily
injections to boost white blood cells, (Garry becoming quite
slick at stabbing my stomach painlessly) there has been little
need for medication – just a few anti-sickness, just-in-case...

However, with no need for extra determination to
work through pain, fear and discomfort, depressive
symptoms slip into my consciousness for moments of
expression: inexplicable crying and despondent thoughts hold
sway on Tuesday morning, until

I have emotions, but I am not my emotions; who am I

I have thoughts, but I am not my thoughts; who am I

relieve the despairing forlornness.

I'm very grateful for such an improvement, brought about, I am sure, as a result of:

Friends' continued caring thought;

Being held in green and turquoise energy;

Healing, healing, healing;

Noticing breath, breathing;

Garry's porridge to start each day;

Hydration and frequency of food keeping body energised and flowing.

Within the inner garden, as well as lying in the soft grass, being suffused with green and turquoise, I've taken time to wander to the edge of my enclosed domain – to the gate that opens up to a cliff top!

It's good to pause and survey the ocean, the horizon, the shimmering silver light across the waves…and to look down at the tempting beach.

Following the gently sloping zig-zag path, I reach the foot of the cliff and enjoy warm sand between my toes…

There's a stone structure on the beach: three smooth boulders piled on top of each other; to the imaginal eye they could be a contemporary stone 'person' – hips, middle and head – unmoving, watching the ocean…

As I look closer, I notice more stones on each side of the three; are they statue's arms? Is this a stone 'person'? Or perhaps a convenient seat?

With childlike anticipation, I ease my hips between the 'arms' and lean back against the stone 'body'; the boulders make a warm comforting 'brace' for me to sit cross-legged on the secluded beach.

My eyes roam the scene before me: blue sky; the horizon; the ocean — its surface shimmering silver; the gentle inward and outward rippling tide...

With eyes closed, I listen to each wave moving towards me...and away; towards me...and away; towards me...and away...

My breath, my breathing, rises and falls...gradually becoming synchronised with the movement of each wave...

I relax, and seamlessly become one with my stone enclave; I am protected; peaceful; safe...

After a while, I take a deep breath and open my eyes; then I'm transfixed by the sand around me — although dampened by the tide, it's possible to discern each grain in the varied sandy mix of brown, orange, yellow...

...billions and billions...

I gaze up at the sky...

...billions and billions...

And wonder about mankind...

...billions and billions...

Today,

at this moment,

someone is being born,

someone is taking their last breath,

someone is exhilarated with success,

someone is daunted by failure,

someone is filled with well-being,

someone is wracked with illness,

someone is enjoying vacation,

someone is lacking freedom,

someone is earning much,

someone is struggling to survive,

someone is intrinsically happy,

someone is burdened by sadness,

someone is aware of who they are,

someone is searching for meaning;

Billions and billions...

Each, affirmed in our thought, is loved.

The love of billions and billions is the purpose of stones on the beach.

And so it is.

Love, Suzanne

'Give me love

Give me love

Give me peace on earth

Give me light

Give me life...

Give me hope

Help me cope, with this heavy load

Trying to touch and reach you with

Heart and soul.' [George Harrison]

Comment:

'Your love and caring for each other is very special.'

'Yes! So much love to you both! And, Extreme Gentleness!'

'Thanks for the lovely message!'

26 Eleventh

July 4th 2018

Day 11 after chemo treatment is a significant watershed where waking up feels almost normal, and each day is not controlled by needing to be near the bathroom!

The side-effects after treatment 3 have been much less problematic, though, as we come to the end of the second week of this cycle, the mild symptoms seem to linger – broken skin on my face; a burn-like reaction on the back of my left hand; and an occasional irritable cough indicating that food is *immediately* needed to calm the digestive tract.

The treatment is going well.

However, I fall short in my emotional/spiritual focus: allowing chemo treatment and side-effects to take over thoughts, feelings and conversations; and find myself using meditative practices just for relaxation and easing physical issues, when I'm perfectly aware that true meditation is setting aside time to notice breath and breathing...no images, no experiences...just because...

'We never lose our demons, just learn to live above them.' [Movie: Dr Strange]

I can't help the occasional episodes of crying.

It's *cancer*.

I continue to feel dismay that cancer manifest in my body, in my breast: 'It cannot be real. This cannot have happened to me. Why did it happen? Why did it have to happen to me?'

Eventually, my rational mind, my healing mind, my rational self, my healing self, direct the energy of each negative thought and feeling into my healing Heart where green petals unfurl with self-love, understanding and wisdom.

Wisdom is deep within; I welcome its expression through every part of me.

'Hey, Mr Tambourine Man...' [Bob Dylan]

Over the years, whether or not there's been a problem to be addressed, I've persisted in a curious, irritating habit: asking, *'Is everything alright?'*

The enquiry is never a conversational question, it is sought-after validation that, however things are, however things seem, everything is indeed, *'Alright.'*

Nevertheless, my personality is such that, whenever anything – even small issues - are not 'alright', they must be *made* to be 'alright', immediately; my restless need to control, to have fixed, to make things 'as they should be', takes over, instead of using wisdom for considered time and thought...

Hence, following the diagnosis of cancer, and during weeks of chemo treatment, my attitude has been:

I have to make this right;

I need healing; I need it now;

I want wellness; I want wellness now;

I am fine; I have to be fine;

I want this over with, done, lessons learned, moving on...

Determination and positive thought are certainly useful qualities, but, expressed in these ways, they are *not* the route towards my healing.

Indeed, my treatment regime must be about *perseverance* and *patience*; to have the *resolve* and *courage* to see my healing through to its completion for my total highest good.

Upon initial diagnosis, patience and perseverance were working well through me, together with the wisdom of knowing that cancer had taken me on to a new path: of letting go of the responsibility for others, of thinking I *must* be active, working, doing voluntary activities, helping others. In fact, the presence of cancer enabled me to say, 'no' and 'no more' where, otherwise, I would have continued paying attention to others at the expense of 'me'.

Healing – emotionally and spiritually - seemed to have been accomplished.

But, as chemo treatment 4 looms, doubts invade my being, my mind fills with scattered, anxious pondering:

Will four treatments be enough?

Has the lump shrunk as much as doctors hoped and expected?

Will the next MRI – a week after treatment 4 – show no cancer?

Will there still be cancer?

Will I need four more treatments, as originally planned?

Will cancer ever go away?

Resolve and courage are not as strong as they could be:

I want this over; I want to declare that things are *'alright'*, that we have fixed the 'blip', that I am 'ok', so that we can move on without thinking and talking about all this stuff; I want this done and finished.

Perseverance and patience have not yet become an integral part of me.

I'm afraid. I fear how much more I will have to go through physically, in order to achieve what I need to emotionally, mentally, spiritually. I'm afraid.

Will I do it?

Yes.

Will I succeed?

Yes.

'We have all the time in the world

Time enough for life

To unfold

All the precious things

Love has in store

We have all the love in the world

If that's all we have

You will find

We need nothing more.

Every step of the way

Will find us

With the cares of the world

Far behind us

We have all the time in the world

Just for love

Nothing more

Nothing less

Only Love.' [Hal David, John Barry]

The last day of June would have been my Mother's 93rd birthday. I think she'd have hated being 93. Indeed she didn't much want to be an old woman of 80 - she was always fashion-consciously young!

I held her hand at the moment of her passing – six months before her 80th birthday, and felt satisfied then, and now, that I'm able to 'walk my talk' about death and dying.

However, I've never held a fascination about whether there is a loved one 'around me'. In fact, I think that those, 'in spirit' should be allowed to carry on their existence without hindrance from those who want answers from, 'the other side'.

So, I was surprised, on the evening of my Mum's birthday, to perceive my Aunt Ada – one of my Mother's sisters.

Ada passed away some years ago, having reached her mid 90s. She bequeathed to me a small brass Buddha that she knew I'd appreciate, though to her it was simply an ornament that Uncle George had brought home; the icon had no religious or spiritual significance for either of them, but its presence in my home occasionally brought them into my thought.

Ada looked radiant.

Stupidly, I asked, 'Is Mum alright?'

Her voice had a familiar hesitancy, yet she spoke with a sense of positive knowing,

*'She's alright. **You are too**. I'm your Godmother. I came because I could...to do what Godmother's do...to watch over you.'*

The exchange was short, but her words carried extra meaning: When her later-in-life partner, Bob, had passed away, Ada had told her sisters how much she'd missed him driving some distance to see her, how he'd helped her over the loneliness of widowhood; and then, one lonely summer's evening, as she'd walked through the village, she'd felt pressure on her shoulder, and heard Bob's voice, *'I came when I could.'*

Ada's visitation made me feel peaceful and satisfied – I hadn't looked for the experience...hadn't even thought about her being my Godmother until she mentioned it, but her appearance, on Mum's birthday, seemed appropriate.

A couple of days later, Ada was in my thought again: without 'seeing' her, I remembered the occasion of my Church of England confirmation, how she and other Aunts and Uncles had travelled to Lincoln, how she had gifted me a Bible bound in white leather...

The thought persisted. I heard her suggest that I should reach the Bible from the very top shelf of our bookcase, *'Look inside...at the inscription; you'll like the date!'*

Yes! I liked the date. 11ᵗʰ April.

How interesting that she should point it out:

Ada had come to be with me in church for my confirmation, 11ᵗʰ April 1973;

Then, exactly 8 years later, we'd been together again in the same church to celebrate my wedding, 11ᵗʰ April 1981!

There's surely a particular way of knowing when one is, 'as spirit':

'You're alright.'

Comment:

'Thank you Suzanne. How beautiful to have a visit from your godmother and a celebration of the 11th, and to have that message, "You're all right!" Wonderful to hear those words.' Love, Alan

'Hi, love, such beautiful sharing. And how wonderful for Aunt Ada to make an appearance. I am ever so grateful that this past chemo session has been a bit easier on your body and mind. I continue to be grateful for your sharing of your experience and you're incredible honesty through all of this. I also believe that all we have is this moment and it is my sincere wish that this next chemo treatment be the last one that you will need. Although we know that being wed to outcome can cause suffering. So as you said, whatever is for your most highest good. I'm holding you in my heart sending you much love - arms around to you and Garry.' Love you so much, Mar

27 In My Room

July 6ᵗʰ – 12ᵗʰ 2018

'There's a world where I can go

And tell my secrets to

In my room

In my room

In this world I lock out

All my worries and my fears

In my room

In my room

Do my dreaming and my scheming

Lie awake and pray

Do my crying and my sighing

Laugh at yesterday

Now it's dark and I'm alone

But I won't be afraid

In my room

In my room.' [Beach Boys]

The room is sacred.

I find it within the 'inner garden'.

It does not need to be described, for each person's 'inner room' is personal and pertinent to them.

However, we can all use a little metaphysical help to find our inner sacred spaces...

When I shower, I spend time talking to my body; it receives my thanks for the way it naturally functions; I appreciate its beauty, and make sure I acknowledge each part from 'top to toe'.

When I begin meditation, I spend time noticing each part of my body; beginning at toes, my thought roams to every part, up to crown.

When I self-heal, I give attention to each chakra, beginning at the base of spine, then just below navel, followed by abdomen, heart, throat, forehead and crown.

Each is effective in different ways, in different realms, and all make a healing accompaniment to the practice of meditation, which is to set aside specific time to watch each breath, to listen to the body's act of breathing, whilst allowing interfering thought to pass unacknowledged from the mind.

Today, I wanted to let my healing thought roam through the whole of my body to assure every part that cancer no longer needs to be present; I decide to begin at toes and let my thought roam upwards…

…before I'd reached knees, my mind had wandered to ideas completely unrelated to the task!

After several patient attempts I heard a new directive:

Begin from the centre,

From Heart;

Heart works as requested:

Unfurling 'petals', it expands its love

And filters out non-love.

Of course it does! Once instructed, healing never reverses; it continues, making its way back to wholeness…

With eyes closed, I imagine touching the innermost point of my heart; my right hand affirms my thought as it rests against my chest... Like pebbles being gently tossed into a pool, my heart ripples its energy to every part of my body, through each part of my body, clearing and cleansing, clearing and cleansing, searching out each particle of disease, releasing and letting go of all that is unhealthy, cleansing and healing, cleansing and healing...ripples move through my body...on and on...forever...

'From my heart

I'm giving you everything

From my heart

I promise you that I'll be there

From the soul

I'm showing you all I feel

From my heart' [Diane Warren]

The following morning, upon waking, more lyrics with a clear message:

'Be still my soul the Lord is on thy side

Bear patiently the cross of grief or pain

Leave to thy God to order and provide

In every change He faithfully will remain

Be still my soul thy best, thy heavenly friend

Through thorny ways leads to a joyful end.' [Von Schlegel]

My tears flow...

Chemo burn on left hand is gradually healing, but its presence brings up concern for the next treatment, and Garry and I are anxious as we greet this week - chemo 4 on Friday July 13th, wondering if MRI Friday July 20th will still show cancer's presence... If so, there will be another 4 chemo treatments, once again spaced three weeks apart.

This summer is indeed long, and hot.

'Dear Body, I'm sorry you're experiencing this 'invasion'; your mistaken cell activity created cancer within; our whole being is correcting mistakes and healing... Time to let go of our mistakes forever.'

And so it is.

Love, Suzanne

Comment:

'Dear Suzanne, Thank you for sharing My Room. As it forms around you, may you and it become a healing unity.' With love, Alan

'We are all surrounding you with prayers for the best results from scan. Big love to you and Garry!' Mar

28 New Mood

Yesterday we went to Nottingham for chemo treatment 4 - Herceptin, Pertuzumab, Docetaxile drugs, with accompanying flush and antihistamine, were accepted well by my body in a shortened process from 10.30 til 3pm.

Afterwards my limbs felt heavy, the soles of my feet felt as though they were burning, my body a little wobbly, though I slept well into a new day.

Today, my thought lingers with patients who were treated alongside me.

Most, like me, were attentively accompanied by their partners and/or family members who became our carers - encouraging us with snacks, reassuring words and loving touches; *always there to help...with understanding...their love sees us through.*

Our treatment, and the subsequent days of working through side-effects, is made bearable by having a loving partner by our side.

Our love is returned, with immense gratitude.

I'm glad that Garry also has the caring support of friends, and that he knows he is loved and acknowledged in each message we receive; each person's thought - with us both in mind - is highly valued.

At *this* moment, the loving exchange and combination of thought is directed to all carers: those who know they are loved and appreciated, those who feel under-acknowledged, those who are lonely, feeling tired and abandoned... May they be surrounded by love, and peacefully motivated and invigorated by the care they give.

And so it is.

Love, Suzanne

Sunday July 22nd 2018

A new mood rises up through me: fed-up with thinking about chemo symptoms and self-motivation, I resist careful nurturance and thoughts about side-effects; enough now. **Enough.**

This isn't anger.

It is brightness.

Letting love flow…

So, my first job upon waking is to order new nightshirts to wear when I'm free of treatment, so I can dump the memory of watchful nights in a sickbed, and be carefree.

I desire to be at the 'inner beach', feet on the sand, watching the tide…

To be; to be carefree…

Monday July 23rd 2018

A new mood helps, but finding 'beach freedom' is not easy…

My body's recovery after chemo treatment 4 has been slower than after previous treatments, although the side-effect symptoms have been much less severe – partly due to the removal of one drug which caused excessive diarrhoea, and mainly because we've become familiar with body's reactions and how to deal with them: for example, when digestive retching begins, we're ready with milk, cereal or bland cake to feed the gut; when needing the toilet, I'm gentle and careful knowing that, since my mouth and lips are sore from chemo, and gut is raw, then anus and urethra are fragile too!

However, this time's recovery has been held back by the anxiety of waiting:

At the beginning of treatment, I willingly agreed to become part of a trial, named ROSCO (**R**esponse to **O**ptimal **S**election of neo-adjuvant **C**hemotherapy in **O**perable breast cancer); the trial model meant that, instead of the standard order of 8 chemo treatments, I received drug treatment '5 to 8' *first*. The trial hopes to show that these four 'end of treatment' drugs are enough to arrest the cancer, and may mean that only four treatments are necessary, rather than the standard eight.

An MRI at the end of 4 treatments shows the status of cancer – *has it gone, or not?*

Here I am...after 4 treatments...having had the latest MRI...waiting and wondering...

And my friends wait and wonder...praying for a 'good' result...enquiring what will happen next...

Today, in an attempt to control anxiety, my mind and emotions affirm that:

My immediate future is not determined by a medical decision

How I feel and think is not controlled by the condition of my body

I've managed 4 chemo treatments...so I'm capable of managing 4 more

Each chemo treatment means a tough week of managing side-effects

Just four weeks of toughness is a little within a lifetime

Four more treatments will end by October

March to October is only 7 months of my life

I can do this

I *have* to do this

I'm learning patience and perseverance...

Am I patient?

Can I persevere?

Can me and my body endure?

Can Garry endure?

I wonder:

Have I done enough?

Is cancer still there?

Research nurse has suggested that the remaining lump could be scar tissue...

How do I find optimism?

Where is my **Ultimate Trust?**

I feel spiritually inauthentic when negative feelings persist despite a continuous stream of positive images...

With a *'new mood'*, I'd hoped not to feel needy...

Nevertheless, not only do I feel anxious and isolated, waiting for the communication of scan results...perhaps by letter, maybe a phone call...wondering whether I'll be ready for the news...wondering how I'll react...

But also, I feel apprehensive rather than *empowered*, especially when I ponder the protocol of the Consultant's clinic that we endure each month; the procedure seems to me to be insensitive:

Patients are asked to wait, alone, while doctor and team can be heard discussing one's case in the adjoining office... We wait and wonder, in enforced separation...until the team descend into the room to impart what they already know...creating a feeling of isolation and bewilderment... Then comes the curious protocol when Consultant briefly leaves the room while patient is perfunctorily prepared for examination, and he returns to carefully lift one's discrete cover... *(It's a physical body! You're a doctor! I'm a patient!* **Why the mysterious practice?)** The medical consultation with a junior doctor changes in style and intensity when Consultant finally leaves...for further private discussion and decisions in that room next door...

Actually, I am fortunate to have Dr Chan as my Consultant – an eminent professor, renowned in his field, he is compassionate, friendly and huggable...

However, this hospital clinic protocol does nothing to bring clinicians and patients together - *as a team* - working towards wellness.

My thoughts continue in judgment, a sense of isolation, and injustice, but, as the weekend progresses, with caring friends making sure Garry and me are drawn into happy social gatherings, my mind brings up a much played song… The uplifting lyrics helped me when I was depressed, and my mind's accompanying images have always made me smile:

'Sometimes in our lives we all have pain

We all have sorrow

But if we are wise

We know that there's always tomorrow

Lean on me, when you're not strong

And I'll be your friend

I'll help you carry on

For it won't be long

'Til I'm gonna need

Somebody to lean on

Please swallow your pride

If I have things you need to borrow

For no one can fill those of your needs

That you won't let show

You just call on me brother, when you need a hand

We all need somebody to lean on

I just might have a problem that you'll understand

We all need somebody to lean on

Lean on me, when you're not strong

And I'll be your friend

I'll help you carry on

For it won't be long

'Til I'm gonna need

Somebody to lean on

You just call on me brother, when you need a hand

We all need somebody to lean on

If there is a load you have to bear

That you can't carry

I'm right up the road

I'll share your load

If you just call me

If you need a friend call me

If you ever need a friend call me

Call me, call me, call me' [Bill Withers]

Years ago, while experiencing deep depression, the song wasn't just in my mind, it also frequently played on the radio, and, each time I heard it, there was a distinct image of the person singing to me: dressed in top hat and tuxedo, he idly leaned against an ancient lamplight and used his old fashioned cane to touch his hat, tilting its brim, in friendly acknowledgment; then, as the song tempo became animated (*'you just call on me brother…'*) he danced before me, tossing his cane from hand to hand!

I was constantly entranced by the image, and played the song to an artist friend; describing the scene, I asked him to draw it for me…

The small commission seemed to take a long time; when I tentative asked, 'What's the problem with the artwork, Tony?'

He scratched his chin, and with a puzzled frown, murmured, 'It's the face: every time I sketch, it looks like **Jesus.**'

...**One** set of footprints in the sand.

Comment:

'Dear Suzanne, I've read your's of 23rd with interest. I've asked the I Ching 4 questions to which replies were all positive, so I'm concluding that one set of footprints means that you're doing fine and can relax through the remaining treatments. Well done. With congratulations and love to you and Garry,' Alan.

'Thank you for sharing so authentically. This experience has indeed turned your lives inside out. I hold you gently in my heart with great respect and love. Yes! Order the new nightshirts!' Mar

29 Heart's Seasons

August 14th 2018

It felt *so* good to have had a two-night stay away; my penchant for shopping knows no bounds!

During the second night I kept waking – not with restlessness – but with thought, savouring the moments and occasionally getting up to gaze at the London skyline across Olympic Park; my mind heard, *'Don't stop believing'* [Journey]

Home again, the house doesn't feel the sick place that I was afraid it had become, and when a friend enquired how I was feeling, I could honestly say, 'Brilliant'!

Now, appreciatively perusing my purchases, my sound system plays Shaina Noll...

I like to think the lyrics are for everyone working with Chemo treatment:

'How could anyone ever tell you

You were anything less that beautiful?

How could anyone ever tell you

You were less than whole?

How could anyone fail to notice

That your loving is a miracle?

How deeply you're connected to my soul.' [Libby Roderick]

Love, Suzanne

August 21st 2018

One of you has commented, 'What an adventure your life is, Suzanne!'

Another, 'Your writing is vulnerably honest, and that is truly brave.'

To be honest, I'd rather *not* have had this adventurous part of my life – for me and for Garry; and, although yesterday, as we drove from Nottingham City Hospital, we agreed that - so far - I've been brave... I could not have embraced this chapter, in the way that I have, without *others, by our side, willing me on.*

Today's examination by Dr Chan's Registrar, prior to treatment 6 on Friday, took longer than normal:

As she probed my beautiful breast she murmured, 'Please could you confirm for me the location of the lump.'

I looked up at her face, 'You can't feel it, can you?'

She pursed her lips, 'There's no edge...it's indiscernible.'

We're pleased.

You're thrilled.

The planned treatment continues: chemo treatment 6, 7, 8; surgery to remove tissue that surrounded the lump; radiation; Herceptin injections. And, as the nurse affirmed, we'll be well ready for our cruise holiday, mid December.

My life - unusual as it had been prior to breast cancer diagnosis - will never be the same. I don't want it to be. **I will always 'love, and be loved, just because I got up this morning.'**

I'll live in a special place, from a special place: from the heart...to the heart.

Sometimes, this way of living will make me cry; but my tears are special tears – of love, and of knowing:

'In a very unusual way
One time I needed you
In a very unusual way

You were my friend

Maybe it lasted a day

Maybe it lasted an hour

But somehow it will never end.

In a very unusual way

I think I'm in love with you

In a very unusual way

I want to cry

Something inside me goes weak

Something inside me surrenders

And you're the reason why, you're the reason why

You don't know what you do to me

You don't have a clue

You can't tell what it's like to be me looking at you

It scares me so that I can hardly speak.

In a very unusual way

I owe what I am to you

Though at time it appears I won't stay, I'll never go.

Special to me in my life

Since the first day that I met you

How could I ever forget you

Once you had touched my soul

In a very unusual way

You made me whole.' [Maury Yeston]

You have indeed helped to make me *Whole*.

September 10th 2018

Here follows some grim detail, but no sadness...

For two weeks, following chemo treatment 6, I've had to stay close to the bathroom suffering the whole variety of toilet challenges: for a few days body struggled every few hours to 'eliminate', causing painful rawness; then for several days horrible excrement explodes into the toilet. I've cried, 'I'm so sorry; my dear body, I'm so sorry you're having to go through this; I feel your exhaustion; you feel my despair; we have to take 'bad with good' so that we can heal.'

I feel angry that these side-effects may have been unnecessary: when I reported awful diarrhoea following treatment 5, the research nurse implied that the offending drug could be dropped, but, in the absence of Professor Chan, a junior doctor was unwilling to deviate from the prescribed chemo.

Perhaps anger and anxiety has caused another digestive problem - severe stomach cramps through sleepless nights. During an early hours phone conversation with triage nurse, I was glad to know she'd logged my difficulties for my next clinic appointment, hoping, she said, that the chemo prescription would be adapted; and she suggested peppermint oil capsules to relieve gut problems.

I struggle to meditate and to sleep; when I dare to look in the mirror I see gaunt hollow eyes that feel tight and incredibly tired; the soles of my feet are sore and numb – they say it's neuropathy.

The 'top to bottom' digestive problems, an inner rawness, make me feel *wounded to the core.*

Outwardly, I feel an impatient need to 'do', a desire to

keep things tidy and under control, to make things 'right'; my restless mind presents thoughts, ideas, doing, thinking...keeping me 'busy', maintaining 'control' instead of just being.

Not long after the cancer diagnosis, after I'd declared a new life path, an image came into my mind - of a barefoot journey, purposefully heading forward; each time I've looked within, the state of the path changes, seeming to represent my state of being: first, a dusty road, then lush grass, a tree-lined path, an oily swamp, narrow walls, open parkland, rich fields...and now a slithering hillside of stones where neither upward nor downward seems possible; I'm stuck in my slithering with no right or wrong way to move, to make progress...

In spiritual terms, it seems to me that, at my core, mind/ego continues to resist knowing 'Who I Am'.

My Ego, my Mind, twisted and confused as my raw core, *has* to learn – *to acknowledge, accept, allow* – that it *is* safe to merge with Spirit Self in order to be complete; Mind's busy searching is an endless and tiring activity, whereas merging with Heart is restful and complete. *Seasons of the heart.* Whatever the season, whatever Heart is experiencing, it remains strong, powerful, made of Peace. Indeed, being *'All Heart'* is the answer to my searching.

As I listen to John Denver's *'Seasons of the Heart'*, my tears flow with passionate joy: for me, the lyrics are not a sad goodbye between lovers, but an all-embracing explanation of devotion from Heart & Spirit Self to Mind & Ego:

'Of course we have our differences

You shouldn't be surprised

It's as natural as changes

In the seasons and the skies

Sometimes we grow together

Sometimes we drift apart

A wiser man than I might know

The seasons of the heart

And I'm walking here beside you

In the early evening chill

A thing we've always loved to do

I know we always will

We have so much in common

So many things we share

That I can't believe my heart

When it implies that you're not there

Love is why I came here in the first place

Love is now the reason I must go

Love is all I ever hoped to find here

Love is still the only dream I know

So I don't know how to tell you

It's difficult to say

I never in my wildest dreams

Imagined it this way

But sometimes I just don't know you

There's a stranger in our home

When I'm lying right beside you

Is when I'm most alone

And I think my heart is broken

There's an emptiness inside

So many things I've longed for

Have so often been denied

Still I wouldn't try to change you

There's no one that's to blame

It's just some things that mean so much

And we just don't feel the same

Love is why I came here in the first place

Love is now the reason I must go

Love is all I ever hoped to find here

Love is still the only dream I know

True love is still the only dream I know' [John Denver]

Dear Ego,

Please hear these words, know that you are loved; be assured that Heart is wise and will always keep you safe.

Love, Suzanne.

Comment:

'The fear and darkness are a part of the whole...perhaps these difficult times are preparation...so that you will be able to show up for the next chemo peacefully - as you did for the last one. I am grateful that the cancer continues to decrease in size.'

Dear Suzanne, I read your account with great sympathy. You have experienced the lowest point. I'm glad to know that the drugs have been reduced. I hope you'll soon be feeling much better. I admire your courage and determination. With love to you and Garry,' Alan

'Very beautiful. I, too, wish that this is one experience that you and G did not have to have. I am so grateful for you both in my life. I hold you gently in my heart and surround you with healing light as you approach Friday's treatment.' M

'My heart is so full of happiness and gratitude for this wonderful news! And beautifully shared with such grace.' B

30 More Than A Woman

September 28th 2018

A wonderfully positive meeting at Nottingham Breast Institute to discuss surgery that will take place approximately six weeks after chemo treatment 8. Dr Kelsall slowly and kindly explained three surgical options, guiding me to choose the one where the surgeon will take tissue from around my back to replace that which must be removed from breast.

I was surprised that the consultation focused on cosmetics – even with an offer of right breast reduction to ensure that breasts will be of similar size; and I was shown photos of similar procedures revealing perfect breasts post-surgery.

Despite listening to honest descriptions of surgery, drains etc. our conversation made me feel that my femininity was being totally respected; I left the clinic with a sense that I was *a cared for woman,* and felt uplifted and positive, ready to enjoy a weekend in Harrogate where I treated my body to pretty lingerie designed to see me through surgery.

'You make me feel like a natural woman' [Gerry Goffin/Carole King/Jerry Wexler]

October 19th 2018

Two weeks since the final chemo treatment, and seven months since I discovered the lump in my left breast, yesterday Garry and I were once again at Nottingham City Hospital for a third ECG to affirm that all is well with heart.

As we walked the hospital corridors, we noticed the sign indicating the laboratory where chemo is 'made'; we paused to watch a technician in the process of keying herself into the department; she turned and smiled when I murmured, 'Thank you for making my chemo!'

The doorway carried the label, *'chemotoxic'*.

'I'm toxic!' I joked, 'I should keep my distance from everyone!'

Indeed, my continued agreeable meditative solitude means that I learn and know what it is to Be an Expression of Pure Consciousness…in all its variety…

This morning, as my music played *'The Swan'*, I imagined each beautiful note rising and falling, touching each of my chakras…

I realise I'm feeling significantly better, although I still struggle with night-time gut pain, slight breathlessness, a running nose, and slight spongy feet!

However, I feel *different*. There's a strong desire to be *'more than a woman'* - keen to choose makeup and clothes, eagerly watching my hair reappear, and happy to take a selfie, even though I continue to be reticent about revealing my baldness when I'm out and about.

My feeling is that I am **glad about life and living; glad for the unusual October sunshine; glad for the occasional cool rain; glad for the blue, blue sky; glad to be still, quietly appreciating 'every breath I take.' I want to secretly, silently love...and allow Love to pour through me.**

And so it is.

Comment:

'Dear Suzanne, Beautifully thought, beautifully written.'

31 The Prayer

November 3rd 2018

Dear Suze,

I have your name written in large letters on a note prominently displayed on a month-at-a-glance desk calendar (yes, it's an old school paper one). The note gets transferred from month to month as the page is turned every 30 days, so as to keep "Suzanne" on the chartreuse note front and center. Yours is the first name I see when I get to my desk (several times a day, as I'm up and down quite often). It gives me pause as thoughts of you become foremost and all others take a backseat for that moment. Sending healing energy to you is also healing in itself to the sender, as ......well, you know why.

So thank you, dear one, for your presence and power. For while your body is mending, you're still doing your good work in the universe.

Arms around with big love,

Harvey

November 7th 2018

Nearly 5 weeks since the final chemo treatment. During the day I feel so *well*: my body moves with ease and stamina; nose has stopped running; chest doesn't feel tight; my breathing is smooth as I complete a 15 minute gym treadmill with ease; hair is gradually reappearing; our meals are now as they used to be before chemo – salads and rice, with fish or chicken. However, nights continue to be slightly challenging when indigestion wakes me in the early hours, feet are 'spongy' and irritable, and I find myself disliking the unnatural feel of silky, smooth skin from drug induced edema.

It's still difficult to believe that cancer is associated with me, with my body; as wellness continues I forget its seriousness when I become engrossed with anxiety about less significant things such as surgery, hospital stay, squeezing into my jeans, logistics of radiation treatment, and whether we ought to go on our long-anticipated December cruise!

Each day at home stretches into the luxury of

contemplation, meditation, reading, writing... It's what I'm meant to do... And it was with much joy that I received the affirmation (above).

This morning as I listened to, *'The Prayer'*, I prayed for Angelic help with each remaining step of cancer treatment, and through each privileged moment of the days ahead, so that my whole being is joined in Love:

'I pray you'll be our eyes
And watch us where we go
And help us to be wise
In times when we don't know

Let this be our prayer
When we lose our way
Lead us to a place
Guide us with your Grace
To a place where we'll be safe

I pray we'll find your light
And hold it in our hearts
When stars go out each night
Let this be our prayer
When shadows fill our day
Lead us to a place
Guide us with your grace

Give us faith so we'll be safe.

We ask that life be kind
And watch us from above
We hope each soul will find
Another soul to love

Let this be our prayer
Just like every child

Needs to find a place,
Guide us with your grace
Give us faith so we'll be safe' [Dion/Bocelli]

As Thanksgiving is celebrated in The United States, it's good to be re-united in communication from friends 'across The Pond':

'What news! I am so sorry to hear you are going through such a battle. Sounds like you have a plan and are fighting hard. We will definitely pray! God is good! Jeremiah 29:11. I am thankful this Thanksgiving that you FOUND it in time. God bless you both.' M and Rh

32 Goal Posts

Garry and I were immensely surprised that, without any apparent anxiety, I made it through the 'journey' of surgery: first, a peaceful very early morning drive to Nottingham; then a calm acceptance of the instructions from caring nurses, including a warm hug, before coolly *walking into theatre!*...

After one night in hospital, the following week was another successful adventure – managing drain bottles and the sight of a very long scar! Surgeon, Mr Rasheed, had made an incision from just under my breast, around my armpit, and across my back; this meant that he could fold back skin to remove the residual lump in my left breast and all lymph nodes from my armpit, then use tissue from my back to replace the 'hole' in my breast. As a result, breast retains its beauty, unscarred, and all diseased tissue is removed. Amazing!

I'd been 'passively brave', was grateful of Mr Rasheed's skill, managed the awkwardness of putting on clothes, and set about physiotherapy exercises with determination.

I was proud of our ongoing success…until we were faced with another shock during the post-operative results appointment, when once again my mind returned to the doubt and fear that had found expression when cancer was first discovered:

Frightened. Nothing is as it seems. Who am I? What's my body doing? Don't feel it's mine. What's going to happen to me? Lost the certainty that I thought I had. Frightened. Out of control of me. My body feels a stranger. My work seems hopeless. Thought I'd done what was needed. Everyone had commented on how well I looked. Lost confidence in me. Lost control of me. I've not done enough. Trusted them when they said it was a 'blip'. Their words were false encouragement… Patience. Courage. Miracles.

December 4th 2018

The morning at Breast Centre clinic had unraveled at a slow pace of waiting room delay; then I was taken by surprise when called to see a physiotherapist; she was not pleased with my progress even though I'd been conscientiously doing exercises as advised; she expected that I would be able to lift my arm above my head and hold this position for 15 minutes

– she used an illustration to show me why the exercise was important; when I looked at the photograph of a patient in position for under-arm and neck **radiation** treatment I started to cry. She thought my tears were because of her criticism, and immediately changed tack, announcing that I'd done well with exercises!

I was not fooled – by her reaction, nor my own: I knew my sudden upset was about the dismay of the future plan to give my body radiation.

But, that had been part of the treatment plan from the outset...

Indeed, I had focused my mind on the planned regime - 8 treatments of chemo, breast surgery, radiation - determined to see it through; after all, the medics had called the situation, 'curative', a 'blip', something awful to go through in order to live through 70s and 80s...

Recovering from the conversation with physiotherapist, Garry and I awaited our appointment with a breast care consultant. Mr Macmillan was pleasant and kind, giving time to answer our questions, and understood that my tears might be because of the challenge of what he called, 'living under the cloud' of cancer diagnosis. Indeed!

However, there's often more to our expressed emotions than what seems outwardly apparent, and we can become upset for reasons other than what is initially thought... With continued crying I came to understand why my emotions were so raw:

The Consultant explained that surgery had found more cancer than MRI had indicated – a further residue in main lump; another small satellite lump; and in 3 nodes in my armpit; he confidently assured us that all had been removed... He prescribed antibiotics for what he saw as a reddening wound caused by bra straps, and added to my confused dismay by declaring that I didn't need to wear a bra! (Even though his team had firmly instructed me to wear one 24/7 for 6 weeks.)

Then followed his 'bombshell':

He thought that we should talk to an oncologist about *further chemo treatment.*

Suddenly, the assurances we had been given at the outset were wiped away. This was no longer the 'blip' that I had been confidently working through.

It was the cloud that I had feared.

I'd trusted the assurances of all medics, and felt let down by the morning's confused messages.

And worse:

I'd trusted the mind/body connection, worked on myself to let go of responsibility, anger, resentment, being judgmental... I'd tried to let love flow through me, through my breasts, through my heart...

I'd failed. I'd let myself down.

I felt betrayed by others;

I'd betrayed myself.

No wonder I cried.

The issues weighed heavily:

Trust; betrayal;

Clinicians changing the 'goal posts'.

What to do?

Trust. Continue to bathe in Garry's love; love each other; love myself; and await an appointment with oncologist, to understand the reasoning behind the perceived need for more chemo. It was important to pose Garry's questions: Why give more chemo when there is no bench-mark to show whether it's successful? Since cancer has been removed, and body is being given Herceptin, as well as expecting radiation, why give even more 'poisonous' treatment?

Together we made the decision that we would keep to the original treatment plan - complete the course of Heceptin, and accept radiation.

The day's eruption of emotions had shown me that *I must find depths within myself; gift myself more extensive meditation to make sure that every thought and emotion that causes cancer in my body is encouraged to turn into Love, so that I flow naturally through life, bringing Presence to each experience.*

Trust, with patient perseverance.

And So It Is.

December 29th 2018

Thought-filled determination continues: Even more attention to body - moisturising, appreciating... Notice, and be glad of the physical activities that can once again be accomplished with the same energy as before treatment and surgery.

Why didn't they say it would be alright?

Maybe I didn't listen, understand and *trust*?

Moments of emotional pain: What does it mean to say, Happy New Year? What did it mean last year? What this? Private sadness about long term plans... Garry's enthusiasm about booking future holidays brings up morbid thoughts: will I be around next Christmas, and the one after?

Tears: it was cancer; how could it have happened to me? Will it return? When? I'm not afraid of death, of dying, but I'm terrified of dying as cancer/chemo patient.

Resolve: I need to remember Dr Webb's comment: *'We know this treatment is horrible, but you will get through it and go on into your 70s, 80s and 90s.'*

New Year's Eve, 2018

We march up Steep Hill to Lincoln Cathedral where I leave a 'Thank you' prayer card: *"Grateful. Love, Suzanne x."*

Yes! I feel grateful for 2018's *learning and love.*

Garry enthusiastically chooses a cocktail dress for me; it fits tightly because there's still a tummy paunch, despite good diet and exercise - Herceptin nurse said bloated appearance is an effect of the drug.

Alice helped me into the dress, '...Because you deserve it... Its tightness will be added motivation to notice your body's improvement – just like the ability to walk up the hill!'

'Thank you Alice! You're a lovely young lady, selling beautiful dresses, with skills of listening, remembering and encouraging. The world needs more women like you!'

2018 has been a year of *Learning and Love...*

I pray that I'll always remember the lessons learned from having had cancer, and from having endured the treatments; and my prayer is that with each day, with each new life experience, I'll be more loving and willing to receive more love. It's what I deserve; it's what the world deserves.

January 3rd 2019

Our appointment with Dr Chan affirms that radiation is the next, and final step of treatment.

As we drove home, the radio played:

'...you are not alone

For I am here with you

Though you're far away

I am here to stay

But you are not alone

I am here with you

Though we're far apart

You're always in my heart

Just the other night

I thought I heard you cry

Asking me to come

And hold you in my arms

I can hear your prayers

Your burdens I will bear

But first I need your hand

Then forever can begin.' [Michael Jackson]

Comment:

'Thinking of you always and desiring health and wholeness and happiness for you. I am so sorry for this disheartening experience. I can't imagine how difficult this must be. I will keep faith for you as will all your friends and loved ones. **I believe in you and in your complete and perfect recovery. You are a beautiful and important light in this world! Thank you for sharing this journey.'** Love, Bethany

'You are still teaching us, as you endure this awfulness, to look at things from up above so as to observe and appreciate the help and support you receive from all sources with grace. Thinking of you every day. Sending you and Garry much love and healing thoughts.'

33 Radiation Resistance

February 7th 2019

Many tears at my radiation planning appointment and prior to treatment sessions; I know that inexplicable tears mean I must pay attention. My body is not happy about the treatment, but refusing it puts me in danger of cancer returning; I don't trust myself enough to make the brave decision to say, 'No'.

Saying, 'No,' is not sensible.

Saying, 'Yes', is inexplicably painful.

Either way I betray myself: to stop treatment is to bring about recrimination, and I lack trust and self-belief to make that bold decision; to continue treatment is to ignore the sense of what is right for me.

I feel frustrated, trying to make myself understood.

At last, after 5 sessions, a radiologist saw and acknowledged the obvious sign of infection, (red, swollen breast, hot and very tender to touch) and immediately arranged for another medic to affirm that antibiotics are necessary; they also confirmed that there *are* other patients who feel the adverse effects of radiation treatment immediately...

So I am not mad, and not alone in my clinical reaction.

En route home, this poignant song plays on the radio:

'When the rain is blowing in your face
And the whole world is on your case
I could offer you a warm embrace
To make you feel my love

When the evening shadows and the stars appear
And there is no one there to dry your tears
Oh, I hold you for a million years
To make you feel my love

I know you haven't made your mind up yet
But I will never do you wrong
I've known it from the moment that we met
No doubt in my mind where you belong

I'd go hungry; I'd go black and blue
And I'd go crawling down the avenue
No, there's nothing that I wouldn't do
To make you feel my love

The storms are raging on the rolling sea
And on the highway of regret
The winds of change are blowing wild and free
You ain't seen nothing like me yet

I could make you happy, make your dreams come true
There's nothing that I wouldn't do
Go to the ends of this Earth for you
To make you feel my love, oh yes
To make you feel my love.' [Bob Dylan]

A new mantra emerges: 'It's perfectly safe to be well. It's perfectly safe to be well. It's perfectly safe to be well.'

Comment:

'Hexogram 30, The Clinging Fire. Doubled clarity, clinging to what it right, transforms the world and perfects it. It is the same in the life of a man. In order that his psychic nature be transfigured and attain influence on earth, it must cling to the forces of spiritual life.'

What could be a better description of radiation than, clinging fire?!

34 Joy

February 21ˢᵗ 2019

It was with great joy this evening that I sent a text: *'It's all done! Your healing thought brought us through. Grateful. X'*

Indeed, Garry and I are grateful to have come to the end of these months of treatment for cancer, diagnosed last March; and today's final radiation treatment is a significant milestone.

I'd always thought that severe depression, experienced decades ago, was my 'life adventure'; but that illness now stands second to the difficulty of cancer and its accompanying treatment. Garry stood by me years ago through that awful time, and has proved himself my 'soul mate' once again.

He's suggested that I should not be 'naughty' any more...and I've willingly agreed!

Nevertheless, upon recently reading, *First Man: The Life of Neil A. Armstrong,* I was struck by the quote therein: **'The privilege of a lifetime is being who you are.'** *Joseph Campbell, in Reflections on the art of living.*

Cancer has been another 'life way' to help me *be who I am.*

During this latest round of treatment I've learned, RESPECT.

Respect:

For those who work at Nottingham City Hospital

For Garry

For everyone who has willed us on with loving support

For myself

For the coming together of skilled people

For the coming together of people's Thought

For my body (renewed respect)

For my intuition (growing respect)

For other patients – their will; their courage; their cheerfulness; their outward expression of mutual appreciation, caring love.

For people with no respect (grudging respect)

I'm grateful to have been able to face 'respect' so directly.

I've previously written that JOY is: **J**ust **O**wn **Y**ourself.

Now, JOYFUL RESPECT has pride of place in my life.

Someone once told me, *"You made a choice to experience every diversity that's possible, so that you could understand the convoluted nature, the sum, of human dynamics."*

I grow with that understanding, and send my love to the world,
Suzanne x

Comment:

'Dear Suzanne, Thank you for a lovely thank you and a great celebration.' With much love, Alan

35 Always

March 14th 2019

Next week marks a year since I found the lump.

As the days approach to what will also be another birthday for me, I feel a mixture of emotions... Actually that's how it's always been, it's the nature of my personality: no day is the same – I can feel ecstatically happy one day, and quite miserable the next, for no apparent reason...

Over the last 12 months there *has* been a reason to be 'emotional'; and, as I appreciate the present sense of freedom from treatments – the punishing schedule, the awful side-effects - my mind finds thoughts of *how it was then*...

Throughout the months of treatment I just got on with it, trying to make it through from one set of three-week cycle to the next. Now, I feel well. Indeed, everyone tells me how well I look! And I think having cancer has made me more patient, and mostly, appreciatively happy...

But thoughts dwell...

Herceptin Nurse Debbie calls it **grief** about *how it was then...*

I can't remember details – like women after the pain of childbirth, I've forgotten the depths of emotional pain and physical horrors; and yet my mind now recalls moments of 'trauma'; I squirm with each memory, and have to cry...

It's wonderful that the dates in the diary are now 'normal' for Garry and me – meals out with friends, appointments with dentist and optician... I find every opportunity to chatter about our 'journey' through cancer, recalling moments that will make my listener smile...and often there's the same response: "Oh Suzanne, you are funny!"

Actually, my conversation is not meant to be humorous or unusual, it is my attempt to process the returning thought:

I can't believe cancer happened to me.

Nevertheless, as the childlike excitement of my birthday rises, and as Garry, as usual, finds perfectly appropriate gifts to shower his 'Squirrel', I *know* that my overriding thought is, *pride and fulfillment.*

We did it!

I did it!

With your help, your thought, your healing prayers, we worked through the life-changing experience of cancer and its accompanying treatment.

Now, as I prepare to make the past year's email thoughts into a book worth publishing – so that other cancer patients may make use of the expressed thoughts and feelings - my daily thought starts with me, appreciating all the goodness in my life; then I remember all who've helped me find this contentment; and finally, I think about those patients who walked the path at the same time as me, and those who take their first steps on the journey, today.

As I write, Phil Collins sings: *You'll be in my heart*

'Come stop your crying
It will be alright
Just take my hand
And hold it tight
I will protect you

180

From all around you

I will be here

Don't you cry

For one so small

You seem so strong

My arms will hold you,

Keep you safe and warm

This bond between us

Can't be broken

I will be here

Don't you cry

'Cause you'll be in my heart

Yes, you'll be in my heart

From this day on

Now and forever more

You'll be in my heart

No matter what they say

You'll be in my heart

Always.' [Phil Collins]

With Love,

Always,

Suzanne

36 No Man's Land

April 3rd 2019

Two days ago it was a delight to visit a fellow breast cancer patient and hear her articulate thoughts that rattle through my head too:

Who am I? What am I? What was it all for?

*She said, for her it felt like being in **'no man's land'.***

No man's land – a perfect phrase:

A place that feels alien: however you try to behave, you feel you've no idea how to be;

A place where no one should find themselves, because it feels destabilising;

A place for no man – where one may find God.

In fact:

When I'm around people who've not had the 'cancer experience' I can't bear to hear them talk about normal anxieties because they seem meaningless – then I feel guilty.

When I'm out and about, I want to spend, spend, spend on me; shop assistants tell me, 'you deserve it' – then I feel guilty.

I have to make sense of the world...of all this; but it doesn't make sense, it's meaningless.

And, if I can't find meaning, then *what was it all for?*

People keep repeating how well I look; indeed, last weekend I walked 6 miles through the beautiful countryside; if my body is well, why isn't my mind? I ought to be grateful; I am grateful; *so why am I crying?*

The emotions that roll through me are – dismay, despair and anger, and I dislike the meaningless behaviour that is mankind…'man' is not 'kind'.

'I want to break free

I want to break free

I want to break free from your lies

You're so self-satisfied I don't need you

I've got to break free

God knows, God knows I want to break free

I've fallen in love

I've fallen in love for the first time

And this time I know it's for real

I've fallen in love

God knows, God knows I've fallen in love

It's strange but it's true

I can't get over the way you love me like you do

But I have to be sure

When I walk out the door

Oh, how I want to be free

Oh, how I want to break free

But life still goes on

I can't get used to living without, living without

Living without you by my side

I don't want to live alone,

God knows, got to make it on my own

So baby, can't you see

I've got to break free.' [Queen]

Your heart to mine, my heart to yours…

37 May Day 2

May 1st 2019

Last year I wrote a piece entitled, 'May Day'.

Here we are again – with a different kind of pain…one that for me has been life-long: anxiety and depression.

Breakfast conversation at 5am:

'I'd hoped to be a better person; promised myself that cancer would bring about positive change.'

'It's not possible to change personality.'

'I'm embarrassed: we've never spent so much money…on luxuries; you keep spending on me; though I really do enjoy it.'

'Don't you ever think you may not have been here? Then what would I have spent money on?'

'I think about not being here all the time. That's what's wrong; that's why I can't 'be nice' in the community; each day's memory of last year is emotionally painful beyond words, even beyond tears...

Although, last year I *did* change: I mastered the terror, even walked calmly into hospital at 7am ready for surgery. *How did I do that?'*

'You've always achieved what's most difficult, hiding your fear.'

'That's it! Now the fear is coming out; feelings erupt...they have to... It's post-traumatic stress with a large dose of guilt – that "after all we've been through" I ought to be "happy"...'

'How could anyone ever tell you, you are anything less than beautiful?

How could anyone ever tell you, you are less than whole?

How could anyone fail to notice that your loving is a miracle?

How deeply you're connected to my soul.' [L Roderick]

Comment:

'Beautiful thoughts, Suzanne, deep thoughts. Your feelings have meaning, even if you don't understand them. Congratulations on your strength. You are tremendous.' With love, Alan

38 Long Road

Once more I've found myself asking the fundamental questions of Perennial philosophy:

What has been the point? What's the meaning of all this?

'Your feelings have meaning, even if you don't understand them.'

This response finds its target deep within me - a place of heart recognition, and makes me adapt the phrase:

*My feelings have meaning, **especially** when I don't understand them.*

Throughout this book I've given particular attention to, *Who Am I*

I have a body, but I am not my body

I have emotions, but I am not my emotions

I have thoughts, but I am not my thoughts

Body, Mind and Spirit are aspects of the Universe, differing only by energetic vibrational degree; I've pointed out how matter is energy, and discussed the power of thought – 'with our thought we make the world'.

In fact, the presence of man's Consciousness – spirit and mind – completes the universe, allowing it to unfold in ways only possible with man's mind, mankind.

Mankind's Presence allows the 'Power of All That Is' to express itself.

To me, the nature of Thought and Spirit is clear, but the *purpose of emotion* has escaped me...until now.

Now, I understand: *Feelings* are a field of energy – just as important as spirit, thought and matter.

Feelings are not a human aberration to be dismissed;

Feelings complete Universal Energy;

They enable *aspiration; to aspire, to feel the utmost.*

When someone feels utter depth,

Then, they open the avenue to feel utmost height.

This is the meaning of my journey with cancer and chemo - its purpose: to be one who feels everything in all its intensity, to grow closer in understanding life's mystery, and to emerge with greater strength and sensitivity...so that mankind may come to really know its own convoluted nature in the journey to Wholeness.

Suzanne. May 2019

'It's been a long road

Getting from there to here

It's been a long time

But my time is finally near

And I can feel a change in the wind right now

Nothing's in my way

And they're not gonna hold me down no more

No, they're not gonna hold me down

'Cause I've got faith of the heart

I'm going where my heart will take me

I've got faith to believe

I can do anything

I've got strength of the soul

And no one's gonna bend or break me

I can reach any star

I've got faith, faith of the heart

It's been a long night

Trying to find my way

Been through the darkness

Now I finally have my day

And I will see my dream come alive at last

I will touch the sky...

I've known the wind so cold, I've seen the darkest days

But now the winds I feel are only winds of change

I've been through the fire and I've been through the rain

But I'll be fine

'Cause I've got faith of the heart

I'm going where my heart will take me

I've got faith to believe

I can do anything

I've got strength of the soul

And no one's gonna bend or break me

I can reach any star

I've got faith, faith of the heart.' [Diane Warren]

Comment:

'Thank you, Suzanne. Now you're going forward.

I asked the I Ching, for the outcome of your decision. "Hexogram 59, Dispersion, indicates the breaking up of ice and rigidity and reuniting. The task is to preserve the connection between God and man. Hurries to that which supports him and thus attains what he wishes. He does not act from egotistical motives, but wishes to put a stop to the dissolution." Encouraging.'
Love, Alan

'Wow!! This is wonderful!! It sounds so cathartic. I hope it lifts a burden from your heart. I can't even imagine how difficult this journey is. I'm so inspired by your strength and perseverance in both your recovery and your willingness to process the experience with such awareness...and share with others so that they may have valuable spiritual support. You are amazing!!' XOX B

'My dear Suzanne, Your last chapter is beautiful. And I am glad to hear that you are moving through some of the emotional discharge of this incredible experience that you have been through. You are amazing. Your gifting this to the universe will really help those who are going through this process. And it will also illuminate the process of going through cancer to those who just want to know and understand. Well done!! Love to you and Garry!!' Mar

39 Take Me Back To The Start

June 12th 2019

'No body said it was easy

No one ever said it would be this hard

Oh, take me back to the start.' [Coldplay]

I'd expected more of myself – expected to find calm and grow more patient with each passing day, especially as I feel physically very well...

However, it only takes a small thing to go wrong, for me to 'lose it' in tears of upset and frustration, with an eventual desire to curl into a foetal ball, hoping that the world will go away.

Even though I enthusiastically suggest more places for us to vacation, there's a niggling doubt that persists in the back of my mind: *'Is everything alright?'*

Emotions come to a head when Garry collects his new car; I'm uncomfortable with conversations about three year service and finance plans. *What is wrong with me? Why can't I be at peace and enjoy every blessing, **especially after what we've been through?***

It's **because** of what we've been through that my thoughts are skewed – I want Garry to have everything, no matter what...because of what he's been through; I want to throw care about excessive spending out of the window...because of what we've been through...

But, I'm not *carefree*.

The sneaking doubt in my mind cannot be spoken: in truth, I wonder why I affirm plans for the new car's next three years because, really, *I may not be here*.

In fact, anxiety about my early demise does not make me live better, appreciating each moment…it just makes me feel increasingly depressed.

I hear about other women who've accepted counselling to help them through this mire; I understand the need, but I have to work through this myself, with meditation, healing, finding *self-acceptance*.

I spend hours just sitting, watching sky, trees, countryside, unwilling to pursue my writing, sometimes crying, *What's the point?* Although, at the same time I know I need to be quietly inward, allowing my heart and mind to connect with Spirit…

Over and over again my thought plays the lyrics:

'No body said it was easy
No one ever said it would be this hard
Oh, take me back to the start.' [Coldplay]

Then, last evening, Garry's Uncle Michael phoned; he asked to speak to me. His words spoke directly to the waiting, empty space in my heart:

*'You feel that you **cannot trust your body**.'*

That's exactly how I've been feeling!

Long before the cancer diagnosis I'd felt exceedingly well; I'd often congratulated myself on how well my body was doing at 60+; little did I know that cancer was already spreading from breast to lymph nodes.

What about now? Once again I feel well, I look well, and have returned to my sprightly, physical self.

But...I cannot trust my body; so how do I know?

How do I know that I'm well?

How do I know whether there's cancer lurking within?

How do I know whether I'll still be alive when this new car's term is done?

Michael's voice sounded firm, strong, supportive and wise:

*'You've been through so much. I know what you've experienced. I know how it feels. You've done so well. With Garry beside you, with shared deep love, you have succeeded through an awful experience... Now it's the **mental** pressure that must be got through...*

You will!

At the moment, it's not easy to look forward to anything.

But, gradually, you will.

Live each day in the moment.

Time heals.

You'll be ok.

You'll become an old lady!'

Michael's words felt like God's words, spoken at exactly the time I needed to hear them. Thank you!

Eventually, as I mull over what's been said, there's more clarity about thoughts and feelings:

I thought I knew me as my body, and had become uncertain wondering what it's doing that I'm unaware of, fearing I've lost control; these thoughts have re-ignited anxiety and depression.

'I'm not afraid anymore...' [Halsey]

Thoughts about my relationship with my body takes me back to the mantra, *'I have a body, but I am not my body; who am I'*

Then, my mind forces me to *really* understand and accept what this means...

But first, I must accept the process of feeling depressed, knowing that emotional depth eventually enables me to find spiritual height, and thereby discovering what is True.

'No body said it was easy
No one ever said it would be this hard
Oh, take me back to the start.' [Coldplay]

Comments:

'Love you!!! Thank you for sharing this. Thinking of you always.' B

'I often marvel at how people -- celebrated people or the next door neighbor – persist after a loss of a loved one or following a difficult medical challenge. What has been lost is peace, peace of mind. And somehow they seem renewed – not the same, but renewed or reinvented – and thankful for the beauty of another day. The fortunate ones reunite with peace. Thank you, Uncle Michael, for your kind understanding and your support of our precious Suzanne.

I see an image of a smiling Suzanne riding in the new car with all the windows or the top down with one of those long, flowing scarves draped around and flapping in the breeze causing others to marvel at how grand life is. Arms around,' H

40 Nothing Matters

'When all's said and done' is an interesting phrase.

Has all been said?

Is IT all done?

The topic of 'what Garry and me have been through' crops up in conversation regularly; as already noted, some people are eager to discuss the trauma of cancer and chemo, usually commenting about how well we've done, and how we 'deserve' a lovely life together, for others, the subject needs to be avoided...and somehow the pair of us grasp the appropriate way to be.

So, 'when all's said and done', is there a purpose? And, if so, what?

Cancer and chemo have given Garry and I the opportunity to appreciate each other more than the love we already shared over 38 years; it's true, as Garry points out, we could have done without the lesson! But, the tough experience targeted our hearts and brought the reality of life and living 'home'.

However, neither of us is any better at navigating the ups and downs of everyday living; we remind each other when we show frustration, and when we're being judgmental, impatient and angry!

What then, have we learned?

We've learned to use the phrase, *'nothing matters'*.

'Nothing matters' has become a mantra that brings us back from unhealthy emotions and unhelpful behaviours.

And, *'nothing matters'*, is a reminder of three metaphysical truths:

Nothing matters: the 'no-thing' of thoughts and emotions 'matters' into the body where it sediments and creates disease. So, I must pay attention to how I'm thinking and what I'm feeling.

Nothing matters: the 'no-thing' that is the energy of the universe, that which I call, 'Pure Consciousness', and what some refer to as, God, **really matters.** So, I must remind myself that, 'what matters' is at the heart of me.

Nothing matters: yes! When all's said and done, nothing that bothers you and me in the course of each day really matters. So, I must keep to my meditative practice to ensure that I'm not sucked into the inconsequential dramas of living...

Breathe...

Notice the sound of each breath in...and out...

Watch the rise and fall of abdomen up...and down...

This breath is all that matters...

Now, this breath is all that matters...

This...

And this...

And this...

And so it is.

Love, Suzanne

Acknowledgments

Thank you:

Garry, my husband, for being by my side, 'for better, for worse'; I love you.

Nottingham City Hospital, especially the team of Professor Stephen Chan (Oncology), and the team of Mr R D Macmillan (Nottingham Breast Institute).

Julie and Derek, for stepping up, with encouragement and care, just when we needed it most.

References

Adams, B, Lange, J, Kamen, M, *(Everything I Do) I Do It For You*, Universal Music Publishing Group, Fintage House Publishing, Kobalt Music Publishing Ltd. 1991

Anderson, B, Ulvaeus, B, *I Have a Dream*, Universal Music Publishing Group. 1979

Anderson, B, Ulvaeus, B, *Slipping Through my Fingers*, Sony/ATV Music Publishing Group. 1981

Ballard, R, *God Gave Rock & Roll To You*, S.I.A.E Direzione Generale Marquis Songs USA. 1971

Banks, A, Rutherford, M, Collins, P, *Follow You, Follow Me*, Concord Music Publishing LLC. 1978

Bellamy, D M, *I Need More of You*, Sony/ATV Music Publishing LLC. 1985

Blake, W, *Auguries of Innocence*, 1863

Brant, C, Salter, T, Mendez, L, Groban, J, *Un Alma Mas*, Sony/ATV Music Publishing Group, Warner/Chappell Music Inc, Universal Music Publishing Group. 2013

Burke, J, Johnston, A, *Pennies from Heaven*, Warner/Chappell Music Inc. 1936

Carter, S, *One More Step*, Stainer & Bell. 1971

Cohen, L, *Suzanne*, Sony/ATV Music Publishing LLC. 1967

Cohen, A, *C6 Element of Life*.

Collins, P, *You'll Be in My Heart*, Warner/Chappell Music, Inc Walt Disney Music Company. 1998

David, H, Barry, J, *We Have All the Time in the World*, EMI Music Publishing. 1969

Davies, R, *Tired of Waiting for You*, Kassner Associated Publishers Ltd, Peer International Corporation, Jayboy Music Corp, Sony/ATV Songs LLC. 1965

Deacon, J, *I Want to Break Free*, Sony/ATV Music Publishing LLC. 1984

Denver, J, *For Baby, for Bobbie*, Warner/Chappell Music Inc, Reservoir Media Management Inc, BMG Rights management US, LLC. 1972

Denver, J, *Seasons of the Heart*, Reservoir Media Management Inc. 1982

Dylan, B, *Mr Tamborine Man*, Sony/ATV Music Publishing LLC. Audiam Inc. 1965

Dylan, B, *Make You Feel My Love*, Sony/ATV Music Publishing LLC Audiam Inc. 1997

Feller, D, *Some Days are Diamonds*, Sony/ATV Music Publishing LLC. 1981

Foster, D, Renis, T, Sager, C, Testa, A, *The Prayer*, Warner/Chappell Music, Inc. 1998

Foundation for Inner Peace, *A Course in Miracles*, Viking. 1976

Frangipane, A, Quenneville, J, Atweh, N, Messinger, A, *Not Afraid Anymore*, Universal Music Publishing Group, Kobalt Music Publishing Ltd. 2017

Gerber, R, *Vibrational Medicine for the 21st Century*, Little Brown Book Group. 2000

Goffin, G, King, C, Wexler, J, *Natural Woman*, Sony/ATV Music Publishing LLC. 1967

Hansen, J, *First Man: The Life of Neil A Armstrong*, Simon & Schuster. 2005

Harrison, G, *Give me Love (Give me Peace on Earth)*, The Bicycle Music Company. 1973

Hatch, E, *Breathe On Me Breath Of God*, 1878

Joel, B, *Always a Woman to Me*, Universal Publishing Group. 1977

Keble, J, *New Every Morning Is The Love*

Kelly, R, *You Are Not Alone*, Universal Music, Z Songs, R Kelly Publishing. 1994

King, C, Goffin, G, *Child of Mine*, Sony/ATV Music Publishing LLC. 1970

Longfellow, H, *The Arrow and the Song*, 1845

Lennon, J, McCartney, P, *All You Need is Love*, Sony/ATV Music Publishing LLC. 1967

Lynne, J, *Hold on Tight*, Sony/ATV Music Publishing LLC. 1981

Martin, C, Berryman, G, Buckland, J, Champion, W, *The Scientist*, Universal Publishing Group. 2002

Nicks, S L, *Dreams*, Kobalt Music Publishing Ltd. 1977

Payne, L, *I Love You Because,* Sony/ATV Music Publishing LLC. 1949

Perry, S, Cain, J, Schon, N, *Don't Stop Believin',* Universal Music Publishing Group, BMG Rights Management. 1981

Potter, C L, Garvey, G, Potter, M, Potter, M E, Turner, P, Jupp, R, *One Day Like This,* Warner Chappell Music, Inc. 2008

Randell, D, Linzer, S, *Working My Way Back,* Sony/ATV Music Publishing LLC BMG Rights Management. 1966

Rice, T, Lloyd Webber, A, *Jesus Christ Superstar,* Universal Music Publishing Group. 1970

Roderick, L, *How Could Anyone,* Libby Roderick Music. 1988

Ross, D, *Your Love,* Sony/ATV Music Publishing LLC. 1993

Turing, A,

Saint-Saens, C, *The Swan,* 1886

Sassoon S, *A Flower has Opened in My Heart.* 1918

Sumner, G, *Every Breath You Take,* Sony/ATV Music Publishing LLC. 1983

Usher, G, Wilson, B, *In My Room,* Sony/ATV Music Publishing LLC, Universal Music Publishing Group. 1963

Von Schlegel, K, *Be Still My Soul*

Walker, B, *I Ching of the Goddess,* Fair Winds Press. 1986

Warren, D, *Where My Heart Will Take Me,* Sony/ATV Music Publishing LLC. 1999

Warren, D, *From the Heart,* Universal Music Publishing Group, Realsongs. 1999

Whittier, J, *Dear Lord And Father Of Mankind,* 1872

Williams, L E, *Let Your Love Flow,* Sony/ATV Music. 1976

Withers, B, *Lean On Me,* Universal Music Publishing Group. 1972

Yeston, M, *Unusual Way,* BMG Rights Management US, LLC. 1982

Wikipedia